WORKING TOGETHER:

State–University Collaboration
in Mental Health

WORKING TOGETHER:

State-University Collaboration
in Mental Health

Edited by

John A. Talbott, M.D.

Carolyn B. Robinowitz, M.D.

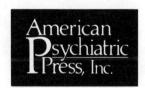

1400 K Street, N.W.
Washington, DC 20005

Library of Congress Cataloging in Publication Data

Working together.

    Includes bibliographies.
    1. Community mental health services--United States. 2. Psychiatry--Study and teaching (Residency)--United States-- Congresses. 3. Hospitals, State--United States--Congresses. I. Talbott, John A. II. Robinowitz, Carolyn B. [DNML: 1. Community Mental Health Services--organization & administration--United States. 2. Delivery of Health Care-- organization & administration--United States. 3. Internship and Residency. 4. Psychiatry--education--United States. WM 30 W9238]
RA790.7.U5W67   1986   362.2'0425   86-8041
ISBN 0-88048-137-4 (soft)

Contents

CONTRIBUTORS

Haroutun M. Babigian, M.D.
Professor and Chairman, Department of Psychiatry
University of Rochester
School of Medicine and Dentistry
Rochester, New York

James T. Barter, M.D.
Professor of Psychiatry
University of California
Davis School of Medicine
Sacramento, California

Joseph Bevilacqua, Ph.D.
Commissioner
Department of Mental Health
Columbia, South Carolina

Joseph D. Bloom, M.D.
Professor and Acting Chairman
Director, Community Psychiatry Training Program
Department of Psychiatry
Oregon Health Sciences University
Portland, Oregon

David L. Cutler, M.D.
Associate Professor
Association Director,
Community Psychiatry Training Program
Department of Psychiatry
Oregon Health Sciences University
Portland, Oregon

Larry Faulkner, M.D.
Assistant Professor
Director, Residency Training Program
Department of Psychiatry
Oregon Health Sciences University
Portland, Oregon

Sheldon Gaylin, M.D.
Associate Medical Director
Professor of Clinical Psychiatry
New York Hospital–Cornell University
White Plains, New York

Milton Greenblatt, M.D.
Director, Neuropsychiatric Institute Hospital and Clinics
Professor and Executive Vice Chairman,
Department of Psychiatry and Biobehavioral Sciences
University of California, Los Angeles

Chief of Psychiatry
Veterans Administration Medical Center
Sepulveda, California

Bernard I. Grosser, M.D.
Professor and Chairman, Department of Psychiatry
University of Utah School of Medicine
Salt Lake City, Utah

Seymour L. Halleck, M.D.
Professor, Department of Psychiatry
University of North Carolina School of Medicine
Chapel Hill, North Carolina

Associate Director for Recruitment
University of North Carolina Affiliated Hospitals Program

Donald G. Langsley, M.D.
Executive Vice President
American Board of Medical Specialties
Evanston, Illinois

Anthony F. Lehman, M.D., M.S.P.H.
Assistant Professor, Department of Psychiatry
University of Rochester
School of Medicine and Dentistry

Unit Chief
Evaluation and Training Unit
Rochester Psychiatric Center
Rochester, New York

Erica Loutsch, M.D.
Department of Psychiatry
New York Hospital-Cornell University
White Plains, New York

Milton H. Miller, M.D.
Professor and Chairman, Department of Psychiatry
Harbor-UCLA Medical Center

Professor and Vice Chairman, Department of Psychiatry
University of California, Los Angeles
Director, Coastal Region
Los Angeles County Department of Mental Health
Los Angeles, California

Scott H. Nelson, M.D.
Deputy Secretary for Mental Health
Department of Public Welfare
Harrisburg, Pennsylvania

Carolyn B. Robinowitz, M.D.
Deputy Medical Director
Director, Office of Education
American Psychiatric Association

Clinical Professor of Psychiatry and Behavioral Sciences
Child Health and Development
George Washington University School of Medicine

Professorial Lecturer in Psychiatry
Georgetown University School of Medicine
Washington, D.C.

Leonard J. Schmidt, M.D.
Associate Professor, Department of Psychiatry
University of Utah School of Medicine

Chief of Psychiatry
Salt Lake City Veterans Administration Hospital
Salt Lake City, Utah

James H. Shore, M.D.
Professor and Chairman
Department of Psychiatry
University of Colorado School of Medicine
Denver, Colorado

John A. Talbott, M.D.
Professor and Chairman
Department of Psychiatry
University of Maryland School of Medicine
Baltimore, Maryland

David A. Tomb, M.D.
Assistant Professor
Department of Psychiatry
University of Utah School of Medicine
Salt Lake City, Utah

Preston A. Walker, M.D.
Adjunct Professor
Department of Psychiatry
University of North Carolina School of Medicine
Chapel Hill, North Carolina

Director of Psychiatry Residency Training
University of North Carolina Affiliated Hospitals Program

Director of Medical Education
Dorothea Dix Hospital
Raleigh, North Carolina

Walter Weintraub, M.D.
Professor
Department of Psychiatry
University of Maryland School of Medicine
Baltimore, Maryland

Jerry M. Wiener, M.D.
Leon Yochelson Professor and Chairman
Department of Psychiatry and Behavioral Sciences
George Washington University School of Medicine
Washington, D.C.

Walter W. Winslow, M.D.
Professor and Chairman
Department of Psychiatry
University of New Mexico Medical Center
Albuquerque, New Mexico

PREFACE

In 1975, the American Psychiatric Association appointed an ad hoc committee on the Chronically Mentally Ill to plan a conference on the growing national problem of the substandard treatment and care of this population both in hospital and community settings. The fruits of this effort are contained in the now classic volume - The Chronic Mental Patient: Problems, Solutions, and Recommendations for a Public Policy. Subsequently, the committee continued its active interest in improving the plight of the chronically ill through legislative activity, presentation of scientific programs at APA Annual Meetings and Institutes on Hospital and Community Psychiatry, and initiation of two additional works - The Chronically Mentally Ill: Treatment, Programs, Systems (New York, Human Sciences Press, 1981) and The Chronic Mental Patient: Five Years Later (New York, Grune & Stratton, 1984). Most recently, because of the critical nature of the crisis affecting one subgroup of this population, another APA task force published a report on The Homeless Mentally Ill Washington, American Psychiatric Press, Inc., 1984).

Through its deliberations, the APA Committee on the Chronically Mentally Ill became convinced that the essential ingredient to improve care and treatment of this population was the improved training, staffing, and programming in the public mental hospitals that still care for a significant number of the chronically ill. To address this issue, the committee convened a meeting with several other APA components who had an interest in this area, including the Council on Medical Education and Career Development and its committees on Graduate Medical Education, Administrative Psychiatry, and Psychiatric Leadership in Public Mental Health Programs; the Council on Psychiatric Services and its committees on State Hospitals and Rehabilitation; the Council on Children, Adolescents, and their Families and its Committee on Chronically Ill and Emotionally Handicapped Children, and the Council on National Affairs and its Committee on Foreign Medical Graduates. From this meeting, several ideas emerged; one, to attempt to upgrade the knowledge and skills of the foreign medical graduates serving the chronically ill in private and public hospital and community settings in one selected state; and two, to begin an effort to improve state–university collaborations in the areas of clinical service, training, administration, and research.

The latter area was felt to be of critical importance for several reasons. First, there is widespread concern that state hospital care is continuing to deteriorate, despite overall improvement in staff-patient ratios. Second, while some areas in psychiatry appear to have adequate manpower, there is general agreement that in many areas, psychiatrists remain in desparate undersupply, especially in public psychiatric facilities, public psychiatric leadership positions, administrative psychiatric positions, rural areas, emergency settings, and in the provision of child psychiatric services. Third, many university departments of psychiatry are currently experiencing some constriction in funding due to shifts in federal research, training, and services funding priorities. And finally, while there are some exemplary state–university collaborative efforts, a great number of psychiatrists, academic leaders, and governmental administrators continue to believe that it is impossible to have a productive, high-quality, state–university collaboration.

It was decided, therefore, to try to assemble the data on state–university collaborations to enable governmental, academic, and professional leaders to see what made some affiliations work, as well as what factors prevented the success of others, and to stimulate discussion on how to bring about more and better collaborative activities.

The first step was to involve the appropriate organizations and leaders. The American Psychiatric Association established liaisons with: the National Association of State Mental Health Program Directors (Commissioners of Mental Health); the American Academy of Child Psychiatry (AACP); the American Association of Chairmen of Departments of Psychiatry (AACDP); the American Association of Directors of Psychiatric Residency Training (AADPRT). The enthusiasm of the various organizations' leaders, coupled with generous support from them, the APA, and the National Institute of Mental Health's Psychiatry Training Branch, enabled the first step of the process to be realized, that is, the convening of a meeting in June 1984, and publication of its proceedings in this book.

The challenge presented to the participation at the start of the conference was:

(1) to present, analyze, and understand various collaborative programs between university departments of psychiatry and state mental health systems in different parts of the country, (2) to tease out of these presentations the themes of what made some programs work well and doomed others to failure, (3) to consider education and training, manpower recruitment and retention, clinical services, administration, and research issues, as they applied to adult, childrens' and forensic services, and (4) to compare state-university collaborations with other forms of government-university collaboration; e.g., city or county hospitals, Veteran's Administration hospitals, community mental health centers, etc.

This initial effort established a data base from which to develop many more effective state-university collaborative efforts, rather than as an end in itself. The next steps must include:

- further analysis of these data;
- discussion among the interested leaders of the appropriate organizations;
- decisions about the necessity or appropriateness of a formal mechanism (inter-organizational work group, consultation process, and/or on-going change agent effort) to expand the number and quality of collaborations, and
- development of further research, testing, and evaluation of the elements felt to facilitate or impede such vital collaborative efforts.

John A. Talbott, M.D.
Carolyn B. Robinowitz, M.D.
Washington, D.C.

ACKNOWLEDGMENTS

As with all complex works, this one owes its existence to a very large number of committed, dedicated, and resourceful people, all of whom donated a generous amount of their own time as volunteers, for a cause which may not have a great deal of status, peer recognition, or glory. They include APA members, leaders, and staff; key leadership in other organizations; and funding sources.

First, plaudits go to the seemingly untiring members of the APA Committee on the Chronically Mentally Ill, chaired by W. Walter Menninger. This extremely talented group includes, or has included at on time or another, Leona Bachrach, James Barter, Neal Brown, Sheila Cantor, David Cutler, Sam Keith, Maurice Laufer (deceased), Blanca Loubriel, Arthur Meyerson, Mildred Mitchell-Bateman, Arthur Neilsen, Lucy Osarin, Roger Peele, John Spiegel, Shirley Starr, Leonard Stein, Judith Turner and Harold Visotsky.

Second, thanks go to those APA components whose foresight and joining in this common cause made our effort a truly collaborative one: Jeffrey Houpt and Donald Langsley who chaired the Council on Medical Education and Career Development; James Barter from the Council on Psychiatric Services; Norbert Enzer from the Council on Children, Adolescents, and their Families; Rodrigo Munoz of the Committee on Foreign Medical Graduates, Frank James of the Committee on State Hospitals, Arthur Meyerson of the Committee on Rehabilitation, Stuart Keill of the Committee on Administrative Psychiatry, and Steven Katz of the Committee on Psychiatric Leadership in Public Mental Health Programs.

Next, our thanks go to the collaborating organizations and their leadership, all of whom are vitally concerned with this subject: Harry Schnibbe, Joseph Bevilacqua, Scott Nelson, Frank James and James Prevost of National Association of State Mental Health Program Directors; E. James Anthony of the American Academy of Child Psychiatry; Jerry Wiener and John Adams of the American Association of Chairmen of Departments of Psychiatry; and Peter Henderson of the American Association of Directors of Psychiatric Residency Training.

Then a special thank you goes to the hosts of our conference in Maryland – Stanley Platman, who originally invited us, and Alp Karahasan, Henry Harbin and Walter Weintraub, who were the very model of collaboration in putting on the conferences.

The leadership of the APA has supported the efforts of these activities vigorously from the days of the Presidency of John Spiegel, who donated his Presidential Fund to support the initial effort in planning for the first Conference on the Chronic Mentally Ill, through Robert Gibson, who appointed the committee, and Donald Langsley, who challenged it to undertake this current task, to Daniel X. Freedman, who helped frame the objectives of the effort and even changed an earlier ambiguous word to the term that we now realize is much more appropriate – "collaborative."

The staff of the APA is one of rare excellence. Our Medical Director, Melvin Sabshin, has consistently assigned the very best staff among these very talented people; individuals such as Carolyn Robinowitz, my co-editor and co-conspirator, who performed the bulk of the work in this project; Donald Hammersley, Claudia Hart, and Samuel Muszynski, who shepherded the first conference; Ronald McMillen and Jane Edgerton, whose editorial and publication talents enhanced our products, and Hope Ball, who oversaw all the steps to support the collaborative conference and this publication.

Last but not least, our gratitude is expressed to Melvin Haas, Chief of the Psychiatry Education Branch at NIMH, who with then Director Herbert Pardes, and subsequent Acting Director, Larry Silver, saw the importance of funding this activity.

All have contributed, and I hope, benefited from this exciting project. Now, we simply have to work twice as hard to make it all happen.

John A. Talbott, M.D.

AN INTRODUCTION TO
STATE-UNIVERSITY COLLABORATION

John A. Talbott, M.D.

The first public mental hospital in America was founded in 1773 in Williamsburg, Virginia. However, state hospital systems did not flower throughout the nation until the mid-1800's. In the beginning, there was little university involvement with these state facilities, and even when these facilities expanded rapidly during the later part of the 19th century, a major criticism leveled at them was their lack of scientific substance.

One of this nation's premier private mental hospitals, the Menninger Clinic, did incorporate both a federal and a state hospital into its residency training program shortly after World War II. In addition, several "special" university-related state hospitals were established in some of the larger states which had extensive academic and public psychiatric systems, e.g., Harvard and the Massachusetts Mental Health Center, Columbia and the New York State Psychiatric Institute, the University of California at San Francisco and the Langley Porter Institute, and UCLA and the Neuropsychiatric Institute. I have termed these programs "special" because they were not "typical" large, old state hospitals, but were newer, smaller, and trained an "elite" group of residents, utilizing a selected patient population, as well as having a strong research focus. "Traditional" state facilities tended to have less felicitous relationships with university departments of psychiatry (1), unless a state hospital was interested in contracting for educational services, or a university psychiatry department was interested in the hospital's research or training potential, or both were state organizations, leading to either a natural or semi-obligatory relationship. There were notable exceptions to these circumstances, however; one of the best-known will be mentioned below.

The literature on state-university collaborative efforts is limited. Despite the current evidence that most academic departments of psychiatry now have active collaborations, little has been written about good and bad experiences, advantages and disadvantages to both parties, and the use of such collaborations to further a comprehensive set of goals - educational, service, research, and administrative.

In this chapter, we will begin with one of the most widely known of these programs, discuss the current status of state-university collaborative efforts, describe several state-university programs, summarize academic collaborations with other governmental psychiatric facilities, touch on some of the problems in all such collaborations, and end with a discussion of the future of these programs.

A Classic Example

One of the best known and oldest state-university collaborative efforts is that of the Boston State Hospital. Its reputation may depend more on the charismatic nature and writing capability of several of its most recent superintendents, e.g., Walter Barton, Milton Greenblatt, and Jonathan Cole, than on any formalized relationship. Barton, who wrote the pioneering textbook "Administration in Psychiatry," (2) placed great value on training, especially for a career in public psychiatry. But it is clear from reading between the lines in his first book that university and state hospital programs were in different leagues. Barton's successor, Milton Greenblatt (3, 4), was heavily invested in exploiting the advantages of collaborations with the university, arguing that they benefited everyone - the state hospital, the university department, and the trainee. He also noted that university centers could not do their job as well if the state hospital did not care for those in need of custodial care. In addition, he states that trainees benefited greatly from a different patient population than what they saw in the university setting, in terms of diagnoses (more alcohol abuse, mental retardation, medical/surgical patients, etc.), age (geriatric rather than adolescent patients), and type of care (custodial rather than active treatment); exposure to more community psychiatric and public health approaches, that might foster more social responsibility; more assumption of the clinical/administrative responsibility; and the experience of learning how such facilities get by with fewer resources. Finally, Cole (5), the most recent in this distinguished line of superintendents, has capitalized on his opportunity to conduct quality pharmacological research combining academic and governmental resources.

The Current Situation

Faulkner et al. recently conducted a survey of collaborative relationships between academic departments of psychiatry and state mental hospitals. They distributed questionnaires to both the 54 state commissioners of mental health and the 115 chairpersons of university departments of psychiatry with accredited residency training programs (6, 7). They discovered that 76% of those surveyed had such relationships; 60% used them to train their (e.g., university) residents; and not one respondant felt the training program would be better off without the state hospital experience.

They described three types of relationships:

1 - Close integration: 12-15%* were described as collaborations in which the department chairperson directs the hospital or the department provides all psychiatric services there. In these programs, the residents see the state hospital as part and parcel of their residency experience.

2 - Contractual: 16-32% consisted of hospitals contracting with the university department for (1) research, (2) specialized services (such as alcoholism, acute treatment, emergency services), (3) consultation, (4) continuing medical education, or (5) training of state hospital residents.

3 - Clinical settings for resident rotations: 83-92% of programs had no administrative connection, but supervisors were assigned to teach residents who spent an average of four months in adult, child, adult OPD, forensic, community, emergency, geriatric, or substance abuse experiences.

Ninety-five percent of the chairpersons believed that one can have a "high-quality" educational program using a state facility. They, and the commissioners, stated that the quality of teaching and supervision, as well as the richness of the patient population, bring this about - but differed on the third most important variable, the commissioners citing close coordination and the chairs, control by the university!

---

* There were differences between the responses of the chairpersons (first percentage) and commissioners (second); chairpersons estimating fewer integrated and contractual relationships and more rotational ones, and commissioners the reverse.

The advantages of these programs for the university departments and its trainees were felt to include: exposure to a wider variety and different mix of patients, services and treatments (indicated more frequently by the chairpersons); more exposure to administrative and public psychiatric experiences; greater opportunities for research; and additional funding for the department (chairpersons only). The advantages to the state facility included: stimulation of staff, enhancement of recruitment, and provision of service - almost exclusively cited by the commissioner-respondants.

The disadvantages to the residents and university departments included: poorer training and supervision; geographic/scheduling difficulties; service demands; and state facility deficiencies, e.g., poor administration, low morale, inadequate onsite faculty, etc. (cited only by the chairpersons). The disadvantages for the hospitals included: disruption and resident turnover, greater expense, and a negative impact on recruitment of those who had bad experiences (the first two were cited more frequently by the commissioners).

When asked how the chairpersons influenced the state facilities, the chairpersons stressed regular meetings with state hospital administrators, whereas the commissioners stressed written contracts; both, however, also cited the assignment of supervisors. Finally, the interdependance between the two was assessed by asking what each gets from the other. The results: state hospitals get faculty appointments, recruitment assistance, residency instruction, and the services of residents; the university gets residency salaries, stipends, and additional training sites (seen as less important by the university chairpersons).

Faulkner and his colleagues arrived at several conclusions. There is a great deal of state–university collaboration that is mutually advantageous, and that is valued by both parties, albeit differently (only 45% of university respondants saw it as "important," and 55% saw it as a minor importance; versus the commissioners' responses of 75% and 25% respectively). Further, successful programs: utilize varied patient populations, research, and administrative experience; avoid excessive service loads and scheduling difficulties; and include regular meetings between the two principals. Potential conflicts exist, but can be avoided by careful administration, specification of their educational objectives, provision of more than just a state hospital experience in the residents' total program, on-site supervision and support, and university support.

Several Examples of Collaboration

From the literature and from other published reports, we have selected several examples of state-university collaborations that are hopefully representative of the range of existing programs. Their selection was more dependent on reputation, publication, and current interest than on any objective standard of merit.

Oregon. In a series of papers, Shore and his colleagues at the University of Oregon Medical School have described their relationship with a variety of public programs: state hospital, community psychiatry, community support, and community mental health center (7-11). Since 1973, the university has trained psychiatric residents at a nearby state hospital (7). The program involves the placement of two PGY-2 residents on the adult psychiatry service for four month rotations, with on-site supervision provided (e.g., the third type of administrative arrangement described by Faulkner et al.). There is an emphasis on learning to function as a member of a multidisciplinary team. While the residents indicated an initial reluctance to go out to the state hospital, in retrospect they reportedly place a high value on the experience.

Also, in 1973, the university and the state mental health division jointly planned a statewide community psychiatry program for all psychiatric residents in the state (8). The program includes didactic seminars in the PGY-2 year; six month electives in the PGY-4 year; six month field placements in the PGY-3 year (two days a week, with two hours a week of supervision at some 40 sites around the state in community mental health centers, substance abuse, administrative, forensic, adolescent treatment, and regional mental health planning programs). Two additional contributions to the literature derived from this program: one spelling out educational objectives in community psychiatry (9); the other, a survey of relationships between academic departments and CMHC's (10). Of note is a comment in the latter that since NIMH funding for post residency community psychiatric training programs has stopped, universities may wish to seek greater state or county collaboration to maintain such programs.

Finally, the Oregon group has described a program designed to teach residents about community support systems (11). They offered PGY-2 and PGY-3 residents on their state hospital rotations, extra supervision to improve their ability to place patients successfully in the community, and in addition, emphasized case management skills. During the PGY-3, they offer a community psychiatry seminar that emphasizes such content areas of social networks, case management, deinstitutionalization and rehabilitation, as well as experience with the chronically ill, including the opportunity to do case management with selected patients; and in the PGY-4, they offer electives in both the state hospital and state-operated community support programs. The results of this program are impressive: after three years, 80% of its graduates have become involved with public psychiatric programs.

Maryland. One of the most dramatic attempts to improve psychiatric manpower in the state system was undertaken jointly by the State of Maryland and the University of Maryland Medical School in 1976 (13-16). Before 1976, there were already several collaborative efforts between the two parties in place, including: training of state hospital residents by university faculty members; faculty appointments for state hospital psychiatrists involved with training; rotations of university residents through state facilities; an acculturation program for state hospital trainees who were foreign medical graduates (FMG's); a Board preparation course for state hospital psychiatrists; the opportunity for state hospital psychiatrists to attend seminars at the university; and a combined residency program. The latter provided participants with higher stipends than did the university in return for an 18 month rotation in the state facility followed by a two year period of service afterwards. Ironically, as we will see later, although 19 residents completed the program, none stayed on after their two-year obligation had been completed.

In 1976, the changes now known as the "Maryland Plan" began. The impetus for this expanded collaborative effort came from several different directions. A new, university-educated, Maryland residency graduate took over the state's mental hygiene administration and consciously decided to recruit high-quality psychiatrists into the state system. At the same time, two of the state's hospitals were threatened with disaccreditation of their residency programs by the Liaison Committee on Graduate Medical Education (LCGME). Mental Hygiene leaders determined that state hospital manpower suffered mainly because of poor quality patient care, rather than low salaries for psychiatrists, which they noted were often double those in the non-public sector, without a concommitant payoff in recruitment. They surmised that the contribution of the state toward the current problem included: poor working conditions, bureaucratic rigidity, and discouragement of academic interests; and that the university failed to prepare their graduates to care for patients treated in state facilities.

The proposed plan called for: (1) contracts with the university for service, research, and training; (2) meetings between central office staff psychiatrists and university officials and (3) more permeability of the state/university membrane, e.g., through improved utilization of state hospital psychiatrists as faculty members, as well as increased exposure of medical students and others to state facilities and staff. They acknowledge that their leadership was crucial, in its positive attitude, flexibility, and high degree of morale, as well as in its provision of good role models.

Two sites were chosen for initial emphasis: one, a 71-bed CMHC, for which the state contracted with the university to provide all physician services. The other was a 1400-bed state hospital, where two recently graduated chief residents from the university residency program began work as staff psychiatrists. In both, residents were selected by the same criteria as in the university program; in both, university faculty were sent on-site to teach and supervise. The results in these two programs were impressive. After three years, ten new psychiatrists had joined the CMHC staff, and there were no openings for physicians; and after two years, 12 new psychiatrists had joined the state hospital staff (30% of the psychiatrists); again there were no openings for psychiatrists, and the residency program had gone from 100% FMG's to 90% AMG's.

The "Maryland Plan" resulted in 116 psychiatrists joining the state mental health system over the first seven years, of whom 92 remained in the system. Eighty-three percent of the psychiatrists were AMG's, and almost half were graduates of the university program. They replaced

50% of the psychiatrists in the state's hospitals and were equally successfully recruited to both rural and urban areas. Recruitment was successful in the state's central office, in the leadership in state hospitals, and in the CMHC's. All the more impressive is the fact that residents, before being exposed to these rotations, were unanimous in their disinterest in such a career (16).

When asked what appealed to them, the psychiatrists listed the academic affiliation, the efforts of individual psychiatrist-recruiters (apparently an enthusiastic and tenacious bunch), and the potentials for programmatic and clinical creativity, and resident supervision.

To accomplish this program, the state tried not only to increase the stimulation of the state's working conditions by increasing continuing medical educational opportunities and encouraging participation in university programs, but restructured promotional practices to reward merit rather than seniority. The university, on its part, contributed by integrating the previously autonomous state psychiatric residency programs and by vigorously recruiting staff and residents for both the CMHC's and state facilities. The new residency program involved six months at a state facility or CMHC in the PGY-1 or PGY-2 year with a limited inpatient caseload; and a year long PGY-4 elective with administrative responsibility or experience with forensic, adolescent, or community psychiatry.

The authors contend that the "Plan" cost the state nothing to implement; although some federal seed money was used, and existing underutilized items were redeployed. They comment that the university benefited through the doubling of its residency program, without any diminution in quality of its applicants, as well as garnering many new voluntary faculty members, who now donate 200 plus hours a week of teaching time. They also note that there has been a marked improvement in clinical care, indicated, for instance, by a drop in assaults.

When the residents involved were surveyed (16), those who had rotated through both the university and state services reported little difference in the quality of teaching or supervision. The only difference was that they preferred the experience of treating adolescents at the university hospital and treating involuntary patients at the state hospital.

Other Models

In addition to these examples of state hospital/university collaboration, several other examples of government/university relationships exist. These include the Veterans Administration hospitals, city/county hospitals, and community mental health centers. Again, the selection presented here is by no means comprehensive but is intended to be representative.

The VA. The largest psychiatric service system in the country is that administered by the VA. The VA system contains about 10% of the psychiatric beds in the United States and in 1975, had 14% of filled psychiatric residency slots (17, 18). Shortly after World War II, the VA began a nationwide program of affiliation with medical schools to provide high quality care for the servicemen returning from the war. From the start, the affiliations were intended primarily to enhance recruitment towards the goal of better patient care, but inherent in such affiliations was the assurance that VA staff involved in teaching would have university faculty appointments, and that VA senior staff members would be selected in collaboration with the approriate department chairperson and the "Dean's Committee" (the body responsible for overseeing the affiliations). Approximately two-thirds of accredited psychiatric residency training programs currently have some form of affiliation with the VA facility (19), 67 of which are affiliated with the most prevalent VA facility, the large general hospital. Over 90% of VA residencies are fully integrated with the university residency program, but there also are some 2-track programs. In addition, several more medical schools use VA facilities for medical school teaching.

Faulkner et al. (19) conclude that the VA-university relationships tend to work well; are mutually advantageous; provide good training; primarily utilize adult inpatient experiences; but present some problems in the conflict between the universities' demands for research, teaching and publication versus the hospitals' need for service. They also emphasize the necessity of: good administrative relationships between top university and VA leaders; faculty integration; coordination of clinical programs; research collaboration; and incorporation of VA rotations into an integrated psychiatric residency training program.

City/county hospitals. Although currently there are fewer than two dozen city or county hospitals in America, in many locations (e.g., New York City and Wisconsin) they remain a critical service and training site. In New York City alone, there are 17 psychiatric facility programs which comprise ten inpatient units containing over 1000 beds (20). Their affiliation with medical schools and psychiatric training programs goes back to the beginning of the century. Two decades ago, following a special commission report, the city attempted to establish university affiliations with each hospital, primarily to upgrade care, but research and training also have been upgraded. Contracts are written between the city's quaisi-public Health and Hospitals Corporation and individual medical schools, and psychiatric departments are heavily involved in these collaborative activities.

Community mental health centers. CMHC's also constitute a major site for university collaboration. In Faulkner's 1979 study of 110 departments of psychiatry, 79% had a relationship with a CMHC (11, 21). He classified them the same way he did state-university arrangements (6, 7): 27% having integrated arrangements; 24% having contractual arrangements, and 73% with utilization of CMHC's as training settings. He found that those collaborations that used CMHC's tended to be located in areas with few psychiatrists, whereas integrated programs tended to take place where there was no such shortage. The trade-offs were similar to those in other collaborations - settings and stipends in return for recruitment and enrichment. Several conclusions that were drawn by the chairpersons about how to ensure quality are noteworthy: for instance, avoiding a monetary exchange in order to preserve independence or developing very specific contracts that spell out resident duties in detail.

Problems of Educational Collaborations

In addition to the problems discussed in several of the papers cited above, several authors specifically discuss problems with affiliations - primarily educational issues.

Zwerling (1) noted that collaborations were frequently exploitative on the part of the university, which bore the responsibility for not having educated psychiatrists for public service. However, he also faulted government for entering into such short-term commitments to university-sponsored programs that universities would not want to enter into such agreements if support were suddenly withdrawn before completion of the program.

Langsley listed ten issues he felt were potentially problematic for training programs which took place in service settings, and even though he was primarily addressing community settings, his observations have relevance for all state-university collaborative efforts (22). Langsley's cautions concerned: the commitment of the faculty and community to the success of such programs, appropriate control of clinical settings by the department of psychiatry, the content of the training experience, decentralization and distance, the identity of the trainee, the funding for the program, a promotional system that rewards research efforts more than training and service, continuing medical education, interdisciplinary training, and evaluation.

Talbott addressed the factors that make for unsuccessful programs training residents to care for and treat the chronic mentally ill (23). He listed 12 that are relevant here: clinical rotations that are "token" experiences; courses that are unrelated to the resident's task; separate (and inevitably differently valued) "tracks"; unclear, devalued, overburdened or narrow roles (e.g., prescription-writing) for the resident; teachers and/or supervisors who are only psychodynamically oriented or will supervise only "good" psychotherapy cases, or who are seen in the university as "second-class" or who are "burned-out," or who are private practitioners with no interest in or experience in the public sector; courses that are psychoanalytically oriented with no systems or administrative focus or attention to functional assessment or rehabilitation; role models who are absent, weak, noncharismatic, "second-class," or "burned-out"; research which is in no way related to the clinical problems encountered in the institution; experience with a "team" where the resident is under the supervision of a paraprofessional or non-physician; rotation only on services that are inpatient institutional ones, that ignore community support programs or community agencies and offer no experience with families, outpatients, or home visiting/home care; and programs that involve the resident early in his or her career (e.g., PGY-1 or PGY-2) rather than after their identity as psychiatrists has begun to solidify (e.g., in the PGY-3 or PGY-4 years).

Eichler, who at the time he wrote the paper was still a trainee, pointed to several factors critical in discouraging residents from pursuing careers caring for the chronically ill (24). Pertinent to this discussion, he cited: clinical experiences that were of low quality or discouraging; the revolving door/shuttling system of care; little exposure to the broader social system; and the low priority placed on such care demonstrated in limited exposure or inclusion of experiences as an "afterthought." He proposed several remedies, including the necessity for the training program to make a real commitment to care of the chronically ill, as well as teaching residents to set realistic goals and expectations for their patients.

In another contribution discussing how to interest residents in and educate them about the chronic mentally ill, Nielsen et al. listed 31 recommendation (25). Of interest to this discussion are those that recommended that residents: work in high-quality programs, including low-contact ones; be exposed to a wide variety of settings; treat patients intensively and continuously; treat and evaluate chronic patients throughout residency; have time to do emergency treatment of their chronic patients; work closely with families of patients and community support systems and other community agencies; and be clinically supervised in chronic care by those committed to such work.

The Future of Collaborative Efforts

In a paper presented to the Southern Regional Education Board in 1983, Harold McPheeters addressed an overview of state-university collaborations with some observation about the future (26). He felt that such relationships were worse in 1983 than anytime in the past 30 years, but that cutbacks in federal training monies would make such liaisons imperative in the future. In summarizing the known studies on the factors that affect the distribution of professionals, he commented on the importance of early exposure during training to later patterns of practice; on methods of influencing the maldistribution of psychiatrists; and on the importance of personal contacts and personal relationships in career decisions. He recommended that state commissioners establish active liaison relationships with academic institutions; stressed the importance of both state and university officials placing a high priority on developing professional training to meet public needs; and encouraged research/evaluation collaborative efforts in addition to training ones.

It seems clear from the existing literature that state-university collaborations can be of great benefit to all involved. They benefit the state departments in terms of recruitment, enrichment and broadened horizons. They benefit the university in terms of broadened clinical training experience and additional funding. They benefit individual trainees in terms of broadened experience. And perhaps most importantly, they benefit the patients themselves, who are the ultimate recipients of all these efforts.

It is impossible to predict the future of particular public institutions - but it is obvious that certain severely and chronically mentally ill individuals will always be charges of whatever "public system" exists. And it is apparent that increased experienced in governmental-university collaborations and sharing the lessons learned from that experience will occur. It is hoped that the literature quoted above as well as contained in this volume represents but a small beginning of a repository of experience and information that will guide future efforts.

REFERENCES

1. Zwerling I: The public hospital system as a nexus between government and the university. State Mental Hospitals: Problems and Potential. Edited by Talbott JA. New York, Human Sciences Press, 1980

2. Barton WE: Administration in Psychiatry. Springfield, Ill, Charles C Thomas, 1962

3. Greenblatt M: University-hospital collaboration in psychiatric education. Hosp Community Psychiatry 16: 167-169, 1965

4. Greenblatt M, Sharaf MR, Stone EM: Dynamics of Institutional Change: The Hospital in Transition. Pittsburgh, University of Pittsburgh Press, 1971

5. Lu L, Stotsky BA, Cole JO: A controlled study of drugs in long term geriatric psychiatric patients. Arch Gen Psychiatry 25: 248-288, 1971

6. Faulkner LR, Eaton JS, Rankin RM: Administrative relationships between state hospitals and academic psychiatric departments. Am J Psychiatry 140: 898-901, 1983

7. Faulkner LR, Rankin RM, Eaton JS, et al.: The state hospital as a setting for residency education. J Psychiatr Education 7: 153-166, 1983

8. Shore JH: Community psychiatry in Oregon: state participation. J Med Education 50: 1067-1068, 1975

9. Shore JH, Kinzie JD, Bloom JD: Required educational objectives in community psychiatry. Am J Psychiatry 136: 193-195, 1979

10. Cutler DL, Bloom JD, Shore JH: Training psychiatrists to work with community support systems for chronically mentally ill persons. Am J Psychiatry 138: 98-101, 1981

11. Faulkner LR, Eaton JS, Bloom JD, et al.: The CMHC as a setting for residency education. Community Ment Health J 18:3-10, 1982

12. Cutler DL, Terwillinger W, Faulkner LR, et al.: Disseminating the principles of a community support program. Hosp Community Psychiatry 35: 51-55, 1984

13. Harbin HT, Weintraub W, Nyman GW, et al.: Psychiatric manpower and public mental health: Maryland's experience. Hosp Community Psychiatry 33: 277-281, 1982

14. Weintraub W, Harbin HT, Book J, et al.: The Maryland plan for recruiting psychiatrists into public service. Am J Psychiatry 141: 91-94, 1984

15. Russell C: Young psychiatrists revolutionalize Md institutions. Washington Post, DC, June 26, 1983, pp B1, B5.

16. Gleason P, Hepburn B: Residents' perspective on the partnership between university and state. Md State Med J 33: 292-295, 1984

17. Ewalt JR, Lipkin JO: The future of Veterans Administration hospital programs for psychiatric patients. Hosp Community Psychiatry 33: 732-734, 1982.

18. Study of Health Care for American Veterans: A Report Prepared by the National Academy of Sciences National Research Council. Washington, DC, US Government Printing Office, 1977

19. Faulkner LR, Rankin RM, Eaton JS Jr, et al.: The VA psychiatry service as a setting for residency education. Am J Psychiatry 141: 960 965, 1984

20. Katz SE, Cancro R: The metamorphosis of the county psychiatric service. Hosp Community Psychiatry 33: 728-731, 1982

21. Faulkner LR, Eaton JS Jr: Administrative relation-
    ships between community mental health centers and
    academic psychiatry departments. Am J Psychiatry
    136: 1040-1044, 1979

22. Langsley DG: Training and service: flirtation, affair
    or marriage? in Psychiatric Residency in Service
    Settings. Edited by Hammett VBO, Hansell N.
    Hillsdale, NJ, Town House Press, 1973

23. Talbott JA: How not to train residents to care for the
    chronically mentally ill (unpublished paper)

24. Eichler S: Why young psychiatrists choose not to work
    with chronic patients. Hosp Community Psychiatry
    33: 1023-1024, 1982

25. Neilsen AC, Stein LI, Talbott JA, et al.: Encouraging
    psychiatrists to work with chronic patients:
    opportunities and limitations of resident education.
    Hosp Community Psychiatry 32: 767-775, 1981.

26. McPheeters HL: Relationships between universities
    and agencies to better meet public needs (unpublished
    paper)

STATE-UNIVERSITY COLLABORATION: MYTHS AND REALITIES

Walter Weintraub, M.D.

State-University Collaboration: Myths and Realities

In 1976, a group of young, recent graduates of the University of Maryland psychiatric residency training program, under the leadership of Dr. Gary Nyman, took over the direction of the Maryland and Mental Hygiene Administration. At the time, Maryland's state psychiatric treatment facilities, like those of many states, were unable to attract university-trained psychiatrists. A 1976 study carried out by the Consultation and Evaluation Services Board of the American Psychiatric Association concluded that, "Inadequately trained foreign medical school graduates carry considerable responsibility in both state and local mental health programs." The APA report recommended abolition of autonomous psychiatric training in Maryland's three large state hospitals and the integration of these programs with those of Maryland's medical schools.

A survey conducted by the Maryland Department of Health and Mental Hygiene in 1978, showed that in the three large state hospitals, 100% of the psychiatric residents and 75% of the staff psychiatrists were FMG's. Most of the staff psychiatrists were graduates of Maryland's state hospitals' psychiatric residency training programs.

Joint State-University Initiative

The new leaders of the Maryland Mental Hygiene Administration approached the Department of Psychiatry of the University of Maryland and asked for help in their efforts to rehabilitate public psychiatry in the State of Maryland. The new Commissioner, Dr. Nyman, agreed to improve the working conditions of staff psychiatrists working in Maryland's state hospitals and to support the efforts of the Department of Psychiatry Research Center, which functioned as a component of the Maryland Mental Hygiene Administration. In return, Dr. Nyman asked the Department of Psychiatry to integrate the training programs of Springfield and Spring Grove Hospitals with that of the University and to recruit psychiatrists for the newly built Walter P. Carter Community Mental Health Center in downtown Baltimore. It is important to add that Springfield and Spring Grove, Maryland's two largest state hospitals, had recently lost their accreditation to operate autonomous psychiatric residency training programs. The University accepted Dr. Nyman's proposal, and the Maryland Plan was born. As the Plan gained momentum, the training program of Maryland's third largest state hospital, Crownsville, was integrated with that of the University of Maryland.

The Maryland Plan: Assumption, Strategies and Accomplishments

The Maryland Plan has been described in detail in our previous publications (1, 2). I shall briefly mention some of its highlights and then discuss its appropriateness as a model for other states.

The basic assumption of the Maryland Plan is that state recruitment and retention problems are due to poor working conditions. No plan which fails to address the job description of the staff psychiatrist will succeed in attracting well-trained psychiatrists into state service. Salaries and fringe benefits are less important than administrative deficiencies. For this reason, we are opposed to bonuses and payback schemes. Such strategies tend to stigmatize the state system and will not lead to the retention of well-trained psychiatrists.

Another basic assumption of the Maryland Plan is that decisions regarding mental health delivery programs must be made by the state, whereas responsibility for the education of residents and medical students assigned to state facilities must be exercised by the appropriate university committees.

We further assume that the university can best contribute to state recruitment and retention programs by creating a stimulating academic environment within public hospitals and clinics. Rotating university residents and medical students through poorly managed state facilities will strengthen their resolve not to seek state employment after residency training.

A final important assumption is that courses in community mental health, psychiatric epidemiology and administration are irrelevant to recruitment and retention. We believe that good clinical experience with the kinds of patients populating state hospitals and clinics and a positive experience in a state training facility are the two crucial aspects of residency training related to future state employment.

The key strategy of the Maryland Plan is the development of University of Maryland training units in large state clinical facilities. The quality of training offered in these units is equal or superior to that available at the University Hospital. State residency training programs have completely integrated with that of the Department of Psychiatry. The two-tiered system of training whereby American graduates are educated in university facilities and foreign graduates in state hospitals has been abolished in Maryland. All university residents spend at least six months of their training in a state facility.

The Maryland Department of Mental Hygiene is committed to providing more flexible and stimulating working conditions for its full-time clinical psychiatrists. Generous provisions for continuing education and for participation in university teaching programs have been made. Every effort is being made to encourage innovative programs and to promote psychiatrists to positions of clinical and administrative authority according to demonstrated ability rather than seniority.

All state psychiatrists working on university training units are screened by the Department of Psychiatry's Graduate Education Committee. They receive university clinical faculty appointments. All state psychiatrists can spend one half day a week teaching in university programs at state expense. This arrangement has provided the university with approximately 200 hours a week of free teaching in a variety of clinical areas.

The results of the Maryland Plan have been impressive. To date, more than 130 university-trained psychiatrists, 85% of whom are American medical graduates, have been recruited into Maryland's public mental health system from half-time to full-time clinicians. Most are working in the three large state hospitals and in community mental health centers.

Rural state hospitals and urban community mental health centers have been about equally successful in attracting recruits. Familiarity with and trust in an institution's administration seem to be the most important factors determining a candidate's choice of program.

During the past seven years, recently graduated University of Maryland-trained psychiatrists have been appointed to most of the key central office positions of the Maryland Mental Hygiene Administration. Most of the 12 state psychiatric inpatient facilities are managed at the clinical director level or above by recent graduates of the University of Maryland's psychiatric residency training program.

As of July 1, 1981, autonomous residency training in Maryland's state hospital ceased. Integrated training with the University of Maryland exists in three state hospitals, Springfield, Spring Grove, and Crownsville, and in the Walter P. Carter Community Mental Health Center.

The Maryland Plan has cost the State of Maryland no additional funds. Resources for resident stipends and teachings have been taken from already existing, poorly-utilized items budgeted for the same purposes. Bonuses, formerly a part of state recruitment efforts, do not constitute a strategy of the Maryland Plan, so that money is actually being saved.

Collaboration with the state has permitted the University of Maryland to double its training program from 25 to 50 residents. State hospital assignments have proved to be so popular that the University's ability to recruit good trainees has not been negatively affected.

Impact of the Maryland Plan

The success of the Maryland Plan is attracting large numbers of university-trained psychiatrists into state service and has radically changed the image of public psychiatry in the State of Maryland. Not only have well-trained American medical graduates been attracted in great numbers, but some of the best young psychiatrists have rejected more prestigious offers in order to work for the state. Approximately 30 former residents are among those who have entered state service since 1976.

The influx of large numbers of obviously competent psychiatrists into Maryland's public mental health system has greatly strengthened medical leadership in the central office and in the large state hospitals. The improvement of the quality of clinical work performed in public hospitals has facilitated the task of recruiting non-medical mental health clinicians. The respect of judges and lawyers for the new breed of state psychiatrists has been reflected in written communications to their supervisors.

Myths Exploded

In accomplishing its ambitious goals, the Maryland Plan has demolished a number of established myths: We have shown that (1) excellent psychiatrists can be recruited for public service without having to resort to bonuses and payback schemes; (2) our best graduates will work with chronic state hospital patients if the job description of the staff psychiatrists is improved; (3) first-rate, young psychiatrists can be recruited to serve in rural areas without financial inducement; (4) successful recruitment and retention can take place without paying high salaries or improving fringe benefits; (5) state service can be made attractive to competent psychiatrists without changes in legislation or state regulations; (6) fruitful state-university collaboration can take place at no cost to either organization; (7) including mandatory state hospital rotations in the programs of university residents need not hurt the university's ability to attract excellent candidates; (8) senior university faculty will consult at distant state hospitals for very modest fees; and (10) curricular changes in the university residency training program are unnecessary prerequisites to successful state recruitment and retention.

The Maryland Plan as a Model for the Nation

As a comprehensive, state-wide program which has been successful, costs nothing, and requires no changes in legislation or state regulations, the Maryland Plan should serve as a model for other states. Details of the Plan have been publicized at national psychiatric conventions and in prestigious psychiatric journals during the past five years. Although Maryland has been widely praised for its efforts by academic and state leaders around the country, no other state has developed a similar plan. Certain skeptics have questioned the appropriateness of the Maryland Plan as a national model, claiming that the conditions necessary for its successful implementation do not exist in many states. Discussions with university and state leaders in other states have revealed a number of misconceptions about Maryland psychiatry:

1. Myth: Maryland is a small state. Its state hospitals are close to its medical schools. With a small

population, it has few inpatient facilities for which to recruit.

Reality: Maryland is the 18th largest state in population. Its most distant state hospital is three hours by automobile from Baltimore. By contrast, the state hospitals of Virginia and North Carolina are within an hour's drive from one of their medical schools. Maryland has 12 inpatient facilities to administer. South Carolina has only one state hospital, and it is situated in the capital city of Columbia, only a few minutes from the University of South Carolina School of Medicine.

2. Myth: Salaries for staff psychiatrists in Maryland are higher than in most other states.

    Reality: Maryland's salaries are among the lowest in the nation. When the Maryland Plan was first launched, salaries for young psychiatrists entering the state system began at $39,000. Since then, there have been only modest increases. Maryland pays its state psychiatrists less than the neighboring states with which it must compete.

3. Myth: Compared to most other states, Maryland has fewer career opportunities for young psychiatrists. This makes recruitment for public service easier.

    Reality: Maryland is training fewer psychiatrists today then it did ten years ago. In recent years, many of the most sought after graduates have chosen state service over better paying positions in the VA and in private hospitals.

4. Myth: The University of Maryland is unusual in that its Department of Psychiatry has a unique commitment to public psychiatry. Few universities in other states would support a program like the Maryland Plan.

    Reality: Prior to 1976, the involvement of Maryland's senior faculty in public programs was no greater than that of many university faculties in other states. Previous directors of the Maryland Mental Hygiene

Administration had not regarded the University of Maryland as supportive of their efforts to improve psychiatric services. It was only when the department of psychiatry became convinced that the state was willing to take risks and to make fundamental changes in its program, that genuine collaboration became possible.

If Maryland's situation is not unusual, why have other states not followed its example? I believe that the principal reason is the following. Overcoming the resistances to change in a state mental health system requires a certain political climate which is threatening to the leaders of the system. The political climate favorable to the implementation of the Maryland Plan was created by the reports of two investigative committees, one appointed by the American Psychiatric Association, the other chosen by Maryland State officials.   Both investigations were requested by the director of the Maryland Mental Hygiene Administration who preceded the present leaders of Maryland public psychiatry.

In Maryland and elsewhere, leaders of mental hygiene systems who expose the deficiencies of their organizations are held responsible for the conditions they reveal. They become political liabilities to their superiors and are soon replaced. The opportunity to improve conditions is offered to their successors. If the leaders of a state mental hygiene system wish to implement a program like the Maryland Plan, they must be prepared to step aside and allow new leadership to take over.

I am convinced that when a state's mental hygiene administration is headed by vigorous individuals who are prepared to take risks and to make sacrifices, universities will fall in line. The present day realities of medical school funding, even the funding of most private medical schools, make it unlikely that a university will resist state pressures to collaborate for the benefit of the underserved mentally ill.

REFERENCES

1. Harbin HT, Weintraub W, Nyman GW, et al: Psychiatric manpower and public mental health: Maryland's experience. Hosp Community Psychiatry 33:277-281, 1982

2. Weintraub W, Harbin HT, Book J, et al: The Maryland plan for recruiting psychiatrists into public service. Am J Psychiatry 141: 91-94, 1984

OREGON'S COMMUNITY PSYCHIATRY TRAINING PROGRAM: STATE-UNIVERSITY COLLABORATION IN PSYCHIATRIC EDUCATION

James H. Shore, M.D.

Joseph D. Bloom, M.D.

David L. Cutler, M.D.

Larry Faulkner, M.D.

Acknowledgements: The authors would like to give special recognition and express appreciation to Joseph Treleaven, M.D., and Donald Bray, M.D., the present and past directors of Oregon's Mental Health Division. Their support made this collaboration possible. This work is supported in part by Alcohol, Drug Abuse and Mental Health Administration grants MH-13462, MH 16193, and MH 18235 from the Psychiatry Education Branch, National Institute of Mental Health.

Introduction

The education and placement of psychiatrists in public service systems involves the development of a new set of relationships between state mental health divisions and academic departments of psychiatry. The goals include development of model training curricula for psychiatric residents, training placements that influence career development, retention of graduates within the public sector, and facilitation of new opportunities for program collaboration between the divisions and departments. While recent attention has been focused predominantly on relationships between state hospitals and departments of psychiatry (1), it is likely that successful approaches in many settings must integrate hospitals with community mental health programs. Moreover, a diversification of the traditional state hospital psychiatrist's role with an opportunity for continuity and linkage to community mental health programs may be an important dimension of successful placement and retention of psychiatrists in the public sector. In this paper we will present the successful partnership between the Department of Psychiatry at Oregon Health Sciences University and Oregon's Mental Health Division (OMHD) for psychiatric education and placement in community mental health programs.

Program Development and Administration

Following several years of discussion between the department and the OMHD, Oregon's Community Psychiatry Training Program (CPTP) was started in 1973. The program was established with policy and programmatic review provided by a special CPTP Board to provide advice to the chairman of the department of psychiatry and to the administrator of the OMHD. The organizational structure of the CPTP Board reflected the interinstitutional design of the program and consisted of representatives from the department, the OMHD, the dean's office of the School of Medicine, the Oregon State Hospital residency program, and the community mental health center directors. The composition of the board increased the opportunity for collaborative planning, negotiating, and mutual support.

The faculty and administration of the CPTP were located in the department. Basic funding for the CPTP was obtained from the state. Over the past decade, the program was also partially funded by NIMH Psychiatry Education Branch, Division of Manpower and Training Programs. Grants were received in 1974 to support the basic training program, in 1979 to support training for psychiatrists working with community support systems for the chronically mentally ill, and in 1984 to support the training of psychiatrists working in public institutions. The goals of the CPTP included the development of a required curriculum in community psychiatry for all psychiatric residents in Oregon, those at the psychiatry department and those at Oregon State Hospital. Another major goal was to develop psychiatric manpower for community mental health programs throughout the state including the more remote rural counties.

The Curriculum

To accomplish the CPTP goals, a curriculum was developed for a required six-month, half-time experience for all third year residents from the two training programs plus a six-month fourth year elective for interested residents. Residents chose their placement from any of Oregon's 32 county mental health programs. Funding was provided for travel and lodging for all residents including those interested in isolated, rural programs. In each placement, the trainee participated in both outpatient and indirect services, which included an emphasis on mental health consultation, program planning, and administration. In addition to field experience and on-site clinical and administrative supervision, residents attended a weekly seminar and received individual supervision with a CPTP faculty member in the department. The weekly seminar took place in the department with a formal curriculum emphasizing all aspects of community mental health service planning and delivery. There was an emphasis on consultation skills for the psychiatrist in the interdisciplinary community setting and a recently developed focus on community care of chronic mental patients. Each year, an average of eight, third-year residents from the department and Oregon State Hospital rotated through the required CPTP experience. Fifty to seventy percent of residents in each class also chose a senior elective in community psychiatry. The senior electives were flexible and included a variety of community, forensic, and research experiences.

Training and Postgraduate Placement

The first decade of the CPTP extended from 1973 to 1983. Seventy-five psychiatric residents were placed in more than 30 community and specialized public settings. Twenty-six different community mental health programs were utilized. Table 1 presents partial data from a comprehensive post-residency survey and shows the initial post-residency practice sites for department graduates from 1978 to 1983. Sixty-three percent of the graduates were placed full or part-time in public service, including VA and Indian Health Service (IHS). Table 2 presents the amount of professional time spent in these activities for these graduates. Seventy percent of activities were in some public service agency, while 40% were full-time public service. Eighty-seven percent of graduates were serving communities in the Pacific Northwest. Figure 1 shows the geographic distribution of community psychiatry training sites and the communities where one or more graduates had initial career placements. Eleven graduates were placed in community centers where they trained. These former residents ranked factors that influenced their choice of initial psychiatric practice (Table 3). The most significant factor was the role model of the psychiatric faculty during the residency training. Other important factors included the nature of the job, the opportunity for direct clinical care, and geographic location. A consideration of financial benefit was not rated among the top factors which influenced initial career choice.

Although comparable data are not yet available, we do know that nine of twelve graduates of the Oregon State Hospital training program between 1978-83 have entered public sector psychiatry, and of the nine, three were full-time in a community mental health center and two were full-time in state hospitals.

Research Collaboration in the Partnership

The university-state collaboration in this training program provided new opportunities for the identification of psychiatric research projects which met the priorities of both the OMHD and the department. Three major areas of research activity evolved, focusing on psychiatric education and administration, community treatment of the chronically mentally ill, and forensic psychiatric programs. The overall theme of the collaborative research efforts has been psychiatry in the public sector. Very often the research focus was on a priority issue for the OMHD, where the findings were useful in statewide public policy deliberation and/or program development.

The educational publications focused on a description of the CPTP (2), on the development of educational goals and objectives for the CPTP (3), on training in forensic psychiatry (4), and on training psychiatrists to work with the chronically mentally ill patient (5). Other education- ally oriented papers described specific settings as training sites for psychiatric residents: the CMHC (6), the state hospital (7), rural areas (8). The administrative area includes a series of papers initiated by Faulkner which explored relationships between academic departments of psychiatry and state hospitals (9) and programs of the Veterans Administration (10).

In forensic psychiatry, our research has focused on civil commitment, the insanity defense, and on the right to refuse treatment. These topics are of vital concern to the OMHD since it has major programmatic responsibility in these areas. In civil commitment, we explored the changing status of commitment statutes (11,12,13) and studied the long-term morbidity of patients who entered Oregon's commitment process (14). We evaluated the arrest histories of this population (15) and compared the findings to the emerging national literature. Another focus of the civil commitment research was on the decision-making process leading to civil commitment (16) and the effect of commitment on patients in various settings (17,18).

The insanity defense and psychiatric participation in the legal system has been one of the most controversial areas in our field. In 1978, Oregon created a new system for handling those persons found "not guilty by reason of insanity" by placing these individuals under the jurisdiction of a Psychiatric Security Review Board. The development of this program provided us with an opportunity to study this unique board, the first of its kind in the country. The criminally insane population is important to the OMHD since they are responsible both for hospital and community treatment of the patients under this jurisdiction. In a series of papers, we explored the administrative and legal background of the Psychiatric Security Review Board (19,20,21). We also developed a series of empirical studies which examined characteristics of patients committed to the board and which explored the patterns of the board's decision making (22,23,24,25). This series of forensic psychiatry research projects has had a national impact (26) and provided data to defend this unique system in the legislative rush to change insanity laws following the trial of John Hinckley, Jr. (27).

The new focus on the right to refuse treatment in state hospitals is another area of forensic research which has important implications for the OMHD. We have begun to evaluate the implementation of this right among civilly committed patients (28) and soon will extend this research to the inpatient forensic population.

The other major area of research has focused on the chronically mentally ill. In 1981, the Oregon legislature shifted the priorities of the OMHD to the chronically mentally ill as the principal patient population for the public mental health system. The CPTP already had modified its training focus to include a substantial educational experience with chronic patients. The research on the chronic patient has focused on outcome of community services designed for the chronic patient (29,30,31,32,33). This work included a monograph edited by Cutler (34) on systems issues and treatment approaches for the chronic patient. Ongoing research continues in this high priority area.

In summary, the diverse research emphases of the CPTP have been guided by the joint interests and priorities of the department of psychiatry and the OMHD. The principal goals have been better education of psychiatrists and improved quality of patient care in the public service systems. The CPTP has contributed to the state and national public policy debate and enriched the educational milieu by conducting research in these important areas.

Discussion and Conclusions

Our goal in this paper has been to describe the accomplishments of OMHD and the department of psychiatry resulting from the CPTP. We described the nature of the collaboration, curriculum development, and early results on the career choice of psychiatric graduates in public settings.

We believe that the collaboration has been successful for several very important reasons. First, we should emphasize the importance of the CPTP Board. The board has provided a structured, formal arena for interaction by all parties associated with the training program, and has also provided an important link between program staff and sponsoring agencies. Although program staff are primary department of psychiatry faculty, there are sufficient checks and balances in the system to keep staff focused on the larger system. In addition to the presence of the board, both sides in the state-university collaboration have paid very close attention to proper role definition. We have maintained a clear split between service delivery and academic roles. The CPTP administers no direct service programs, and the OMHD works closely with us in all matters of psychiatric education and in many areas of psychiatric research. Opportunities have existed in the course of the past decade that blur these roles and confuse service and education. With each challenge we have attempted to focus consistently on a clear separation of role definition. Another factor in the success of the past decade can be attributed to stability of key administrators in the system. There have been two directors of the CPTP and of the OMHD in the past ten years, and the original directors of both programs have remained in key positions in relation to the CPTP. A less stable system certainly would effect the transferability of this model.

In addition to administrative issues, we are, of course, extremely interested in the factors that influenced the initial career choice of our graduates. While the current national priority emphasizing state hospital placement is important, it should not overlook the importance of specific curricular influence on community mental health program career placement. In fact, we feel that a comprehensive model of psychiatric education for the public sector should involve a combination of state hospital and community mental health program placements. We agree with Knesper's (35) conclusions about state hospital placement of psychiatrists and the desirability of developing broader networks of mental health delivery including community programs in an effort to retain psychiatrists in these public settings. The curriculum in Oregon gives attention to community consultation skills and not just to the consultation/liaison role of psychiatrists in hospital settings as currently advocated by many psychiatric educators. This is essential in view of the manpower findings that part-time consultation activity (much of it in the community) increased from 40 to 70% for all psychiatrists between 1965 and 1980 (36).

Finally, the collaboration between the OMHD and the department provided an opportunity for a series of productive research investigations in areas of psychiatric education and administration, care of chronic patients, and forensic psychiatry. These areas are significant priorities for the OMHD and are a central academic mission of the CPTP. It seems likely that primary faculty role models who also are active in community psychiatry research contribute to the credibility of these roles and influence the resident's career decision.

TABLE 1
INITIAL POST-GRADUATE PRACTICE OF RESIDENTS
1978 – 1983

Practice Type	No.	%
CMHC Only	7	24
CMHC/Private Practice	6	20
CMHC/VA	1	3
CMHC/HMO	1	3
VA Only	2	7
VA/Private Practice	2	7
University Only	3	10
State Hospital Only	1	3
HMO Only	1	3
Private Practice Only	5	17
Indian Health Service	1	3
TOTALS	**30**	**100**

TABLE 2
INITIAL POST-GRADUATE ACTIVITY OF RESIDENTS
1978 - 1983

Activity*	No.	%
Some Public Service (CMHC, VA, SH, IHS)	21	70
Full-time Public Service	12	40
Some Private Practice	13	43
Full-time Private Practice	5	17
Some Academics	8	27
Full-time Academics	3	10
Practicing in Northwest	26	87

*Since some people have multiple roles, total is greater than 100%

TABLE 3
RANKED FACTORS THAT INFLUENCED CHOICE
OF INITIAL PSYCHIATRIC PRACTICE
27 OREGON RESIDENTS
1975 – 1983

1. <u>Role models</u> (Psychiatrists or other professinals who became models for career development during residency)

2. <u>Nature of job</u> (Opportunities for preferred professional activities and interests)

3. <u>Clinical care</u> (Direct clinical experience in residency)

4. <u>Geographical location</u> (Part of the country; urban/rural, etc.)

5. <u>Place of employment</u> (Attractiveness and convenience of the place of work)

6. <u>Classroom work</u> (Seminars, reading, lectures in residency)

7. <u>Colleagues</u> (Fellow workers with whom associated)

8. <u>Non-clinical experiences</u> (Direct non-clinical experiences in residency such as research or administration)

9. <u>Financial benefits</u> (Salary and fringe benefits)

10. <u>Other factors</u>

11. <u>Service obligations</u> (Military, PHS)

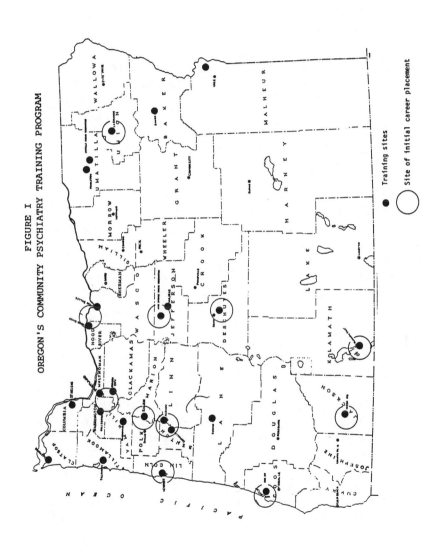

FIGURE I

OREGON'S COMMUNITY PSYCHIATRY TRAINING PROGRAM

● Training sites

● Site of initial career placement

REFERENCES

1. Weintraub W, Harbin HT, Brook J, et al: The Maryland plan for recruiting psychiatrists into public service. Am J Psychiatry 141:91-94, 1984

2. Shore JH: Community psychiatry in Oregon: State participation. J Med Educ 50:1067-1068, 1975

3. Shore JH, Kinzie JD, Bloom JD: Required educational objectives in community psychiatry. Am J Psychiatry 136:193-195, 1979

4. Bloom JD, Kinzie JD, Shore JH: Residency curriculum in forensic psychiatry. Am J Psychiatry 137:730-732, 1980

5. Cutler DL, Bloom JD, Shore JH: Training psychiatrists to work with community support systems for chronically mentally ill persons. Am J Psychiatry 138:98-101, 1981

6. Faulkner LR, Eaton JS Jr, Bloom JD, et al: The CMHC as a setting for residency education. Community Ment Health J 18:3-10, 1982

7. Faulkner LR, Rankin RM, Eaton JS Jr, et al: The state hospital as a setting for residency education. Psychiatr Education 7:153-166, 1983

8. Kofoed L, Cutler DL: Issues in rural community psychiatry training, in Training Professionals for Rural Mental Health. Edited by Dengerink HA, Cross HJ. Lincoln, University of Nebraska Press, 1982

9. Faulkner LR, Eaton JS Jr, Rankin RM: Administrative relationships between state hospitals and academic psychiatry departments. Am J Psychiatry 140:898-901, 1983

10. Faulkner LR, Rankin RM, Eaton JS Jr, et al: The VA psychiatry service as a setting for residency education. Am J Psychiatry 141: 960-965, 1984

11. Shore JH: Commitment process for psychiatric patients – changing status in the western states. West J Med 128:207-211, 1978

12. Bloom JD, Shore JH, Treleaven J: Oregon's civil commitment statute; Stone's "thank-you theory"— judicial survey. J Psychiatry Law 7:381-389, 1979

13. Faulkner LR, Bloom JD, Kundahl-Stanley K: The effects of a new involuntary commitment law: expectations and realities. Bull Am Acad Psychiatry Law 10:249-259, 1982

14. Shore JH, Breakey W, Arvidson B: Morbidity and mortality in the commitment process. Arch Gen Psychiatry 38:930-934, 1981

15. Bloom JD, Shore JH, Arvidson B: Local variations in arrests of psychiatric patients. Bull Am Acad Psychiatry Law 9:203-209, 1981

16. Badger MJ, Shore JH: Psychiatric and nonmedical decisions on commitment. Am J Psychiatry 137:367-369, 1980

17. Faulkner LR, Bloom JD, Resnick MR, et al: Local variations in the civil commitment process. Bull Am Acad Psychiatry Law 11:5-15, 1983

18. Faulkner LR, Bloom JD, Stern TO: Rural civil commitment. Bull Am Acad Psychiatry Law 12: 359-371, 1984

19. Bloom JL, Bloom JD: Disposition of insanity defense cases in Oregon. Bull Am Acad Psychiatry Law 9:93-99, 1981

20. Rogers JL, Bloom JD, Manson SM: State's insanity defense, an alternative form of sentence. Oregon State Bar Bulletin, July 1982, pp 4-6

21. Rogers JL, Bloom JD, Manson SM: Oregon's reform of the insanity defense system. Hosp Community Psychiatry 33:1022-1023, 1982

22. Rogers JL, Bloom JD: Characteristics of persons committed to Oregon's psychiatric security review board.   Bull Am Acad Psychiatry Law 10:155–165, 1982

23. Bloom JD, Rogers JL, Manson SM: After Oregon's insanity defense: a comparison of conditional release and hospitalization. Int J Law Psychiatry 4:391–402, 1982

24. Rogers JL, Bloom JD, Manson SM: Insanity defenses: contested or conceded? Am J Psychiatry 141:885–888, 1984

25. Rogers JL, Sack WH, Bloom JD, et al: Women in Oregon's insanity defense system. J Psychiatry Law (in press)

26. American Psychiatric Association Statement on the Insanity Defense. Am J Psychiatry 140:681–688, 1983

27. Rogers JL, Bloom JD, Manson SM: Oregon's new insanity defense system: a review of the first five years, 1978 to 1982. Bull Am Acad Psychiatry Law 12: 383–402, 1984

28. Bloom JD, Faulkner LR, Holm VM, et al: An empirical view of patients exercising their right to refuse treatment. Int J Law Psychiatry, 7: 315–328, 1984

29. Cutler DL: Volunteer support networks for chronic patients,   in Community Support Systems for the Long-term Patient: New Directions for Mental Health Services, vol 2.   Edited by Stein LI. San Francisco, Jossey Bass, 1979

30. Cutler DL, Terwilliger WB, Faulkner LR, et al: Disseminating the LINC: principles of a community support program. Hosp Community Psychiatry 35:51–55, 1984

31. Faulkner LR, Terwilliger WB, Cutler DL: Productive activities for the chronic patient. Community Ment Health J 20: 109–122, 1984

32. Cutler DL: Networks, part III, community treatment, in The Chronic Mental Patient: Five Years Later. Edited by Talbott JA. Orlando, Grune & Stratton, 1984

33. Faulkner LR, McFarland BH, Larch BB, et al: Small group work therapy for the chronic mentally ill: a 10-year follow-up. Hosp Community Psychiatry 37: 273-279, 1986

34. Cutler DL (ed): Effective Aftercare for the 1980's. New Directions for Mental Health Services, vol 19. San Francisco, Jossey-Bass, 1983

35. Knespers DJ, Hirtle SC: Strategies to attract psychiatrists to state mental hospital work. Arch Gen Psychiatry 38:1135-1140, 1981

36. Fenton WS, Leaf PJ, Moran NL, et al: Trends in psychiatric practice, 1965-1980. Am J Psychiatry 141:346-351, 1984

A WORKING MODEL PROGRAM IN LINKING ACADEMIC AND STATE SERVICE AGENCIES IN PSYCHIATRIC RESIDENCY TRAINING IN NORTH CAROLINA

Preston A. Walker, M.D.

Seymour L. Halleck, M.D.

For almost a decade, the University of North Carolina Affiliated Hospitals Residency Training Program in Psychiatry has integrated psychiatric education into a service base. This integration was largely accomplished by merging two fully approved and longstanding residency education programs in psychiatry and child psychiatry: one in a 700 bed regional state mental hospital and the other in a university medical center. We are convinced that the merger has improved both training and service. Training has benefited by easier and better recruitment and by broadening the variety of learning experiences. At the same time, more and better trained psychiatrists are now committed to working with state hospital patients.

Background

In 1973, a group of key professionals from the Department of Psychiatry at the University of North Carolina School of Medicine in Chapel Hill, the Residency Training Program at Dorothea Dix Hospital in Raleigh, and the Division of Mental Health Services of the North Carolina Department of Human Resources met to discuss problems involving recent or impending crisis events in psychiatric manpower and training in the state. Some of these crisis events were: 1) the reduction of federal funds for psychiatric residency training programs; 2) the increasing dependence of state hospitals on immigrating foreign medical graduates, with the likelihood that immigration soon would be curtailed by the Immigration-Naturalization Service; 3) the increasing difficulties encountered by public mental health systems in recruitment and retention of quality residents and psychiatric staff; and 4) the need for a broadening of clinical training and research opportunities for residents and medical students in the medical school setting. After much consideration of the pros and cons concerned in the proposed merger of the two programs, it seemed to the group that the advantages outweighed the disadvantages.

The reasons for this conclusion were:

1. The Dorothea Dix Hospital program offered a large amount of hard state monies but was unable to recruit quality resident applicants; the Department of Psychiatry could recruit quality applicants but was losing federal stipends.

2. The medical school increased its student enrollment to 160 per year, thereby necessitating the need for
increased numbers of training sites and increased numbers
of faculty and resident psychiatrists for teaching and
supervision of clinical clerks in psychiatry.

3. The university needed an increase in the number
of psychiatric research beds and patients which could be
provided by the state hospital.

4. The state hospital program needed increased
exposure of residents to outpatient experiences,
consultation-liaison services, student mental health, and
neurology services which could be provided by the
university.

5. The university residents needed a broader
exposure to chronically mentally ill patients.

The merger seemed to be timely. Its implementation, however, posed the following problems:

1. Two fully accredited residency training programs
in adult and child psychiatry were separately funded by
NIMH grants. Did we stand to lose one of these grants and
thereby lose even more already scarce federal dollars?

2. How would residents already enrolled in the state
hospital program be accepted into the combined program?

3. How could we improve acceptance by combined
residents of supervision by some of the state hospital
psychiatrists with little or no previous experience in
teaching?

4. How could we overcome the territorial resistance
of the staff of both hospitals to the proposed merger?

We addressed the first question by consultation with
Dr. Melvyn Haas at the National Institute of Mental Health
who, with the concurrence of the AMA Council on Medical
Education, and the Residency Review Committee in
Psychiatry proposed a phasing-out over a three-year period
of individual accreditation and a similar phasing-out over
three years of both grants. He suggested that we then
rewrite a renewal grant at the end of three years,
incorporating both training sites.

We addressed the second question similarily; that is,
we conjointly managed for three years the two individual
programs as if they were one program. The two training
directors became co-directors, conjointly chairing the
training committee and managing curriculum design and
implementation, clinical assignments, and evaluation. The
two institutions negotiated a contract sharing the expenses

of resident supervision, resident stipends, travel cost, teaching costs, etc., on an equitable basis. Dorothea Dix Hospital paid for 15 resident stipends and four child fellow stipends. North Carolina Memorial Hospital paid for 30 resident stipends and four child fellow stipends. Expenses for Grand Rounds speakers and travel for supervisors and consultants between the two institutions also were shared. Residents at Dorothea Dix Hospital were given the option of continuing in the old program until graduation at a higher stipend, or applying to the merged program at a lower stipend. It was also agreed by the training committee that when the old Dorothea Dix program was fully phased out, all residents would receive the same stipends and all residents would rotate through inpatient services at Dorothea Dix and North Carolina Memorial Hospitals without exception.

The third question regarding combined resident acceptance of less-qualified supervisors was addressed by asking state hospital staff interested in teaching to volunteer to serve on the admission ward where residents were concentrated. The environment was enriched likewise by volunteers from each institution agreeing to chair diagnostic and treatment conferences at the other institution. An accredited continuing medical education program was instituted at Dorothea Dix Hospital, aimed towards improving psychiatric knowledge and teaching skills, and a supervisory seminar was required for clinical appointments by the state hospital staff. Staff were encouraged to aim for board certification, and merit increments were prioritized based on excellence in teaching and board certification.

Territorial resistance to the merger was a much more difficult question. Both institutions reacted as might be predicted. University faculty were afraid residents would be inundated with service needs from the state hospital, and, at times, fostered mini-crises within the training committee regarding limits on numbers of patients, night call, and quality of supervision and attendings. The state hospital staff were afraid the university faculty would take over the teaching, leaving the staff to perform the bulk of patient care and creating a two-class faculty.

This resistence went through three distinct phases similarly seen in marriages: 1) the era of great expectations (or the honeymoon); 2) the era of mutual disappointment (or, the honeymoon's over); and 3) the era of mutual respectability (or settling down to married life).

The Honeymoon (very brief)

Fantasies of full clinical professorship or at least associate professorship abounded amongst all Dorothea Dix staff. Other fantasies of visiting University of North Carolina faculty were that they could greatly increase their income by teaching and consultation to the clinical faculty at Dix.

The Honeymoon's Over

This disquieting period was ushered in when a number of Dorothea Dix's residents were accepted into the merged program or graduated, thus drastically reducing the numbers available for night call at Dix. The Dix staff had to take residents' call duty rather than administrative call. Needless to say, this was an unpopular experience. Faculty at the two institutions then began to have heated arguments over how much time residents should spend in various services at Dix versus Memorial Hospital. Faculty and staff were openly mistrustful and, at times, even hostile towards each other regarding issues such as case loads at the two institutions or quality of supervision.

The "call" problem was resolved by using monies saved from the reduction of stipends at Dix to hire senior residents to take call along with first year residents at Dorothea Dix. This solution was approved by the training committee and sanctioned by the university house staff office as an "approved extracurricular professional activity." Territorial issues were resolved much more slowly. One important symbolic measure was to insist that Grand Rounds and some other major conference be presented by staff and visiting lecturers at both institutions during the same day. This plan plus other administrative decisions which emphasized the equal importance of both institutions also held yearly retreats with key resident, faculty, and hospital staff to address progress and impediments.

After three years of the co-training directors systematically addressing each issue, and with the solid support of Dr. Granville Tolley, Director of Dorothea Dix Hospital, and Dr. Thomas Curtis, Chairman of the

Department of Psychiatry, the third phase of <u>mutual respectability</u> slowly began to emerge. Residents began to see the marriage as solid, and after graduation joined the staff of both Dorothea Dix Hospital and North Carolina Memorial Hospital, thereby steadily enhancing the quality of teaching of residents and medical students. Medical students who had taken clerkships at Dix began to see this experience as positive, and applications to the program increased.

In 1976, the structure of the residency committee was streamlined. Dr. Walker, a previous co-director, became the sole director. Dr. Halleck, a previous co-director, became the associate director for recruitment. Assistant training directors were appointed for each year and for child psychiatry. The training committee now consisted of training coordinators from each year level, resident representatives from each year level, the child training director, the training and associate training director, the chief resident, and the chairman of the residents' group and a child fellow representative. By this time, the residency program had been extended to four years of training and had grown to 60 residents. The University of North Carolina Memorial Hospital now contributed 42 resident and fellow stipends, and Dix contributed 19 resident and fellow stipends. Residents now no longer saw the program as a dual one but as one entity. Staff were now slowly agreeing with this perception after seeing some of the results of improved quality of resident application and education.

The Bottom Line

Of the 108 graduates since the merger in 1974, 68 have remained in North Carolina; 51 have been employed by North Carolina public mental hospitals or community mental health centers for one or more years; six of the graduates that left the state have returned. Since the merger in 1974, 16 of the graduates have joined the general psychiatric and child psychiatric staff at Dorothea Dix Hospital with clinical appointments at the university; and 13 of the graduates have joined the faculty at the University of North Carolina School of Medicine Department of Psychiatry. At the time of our last graduation, seven of the staff working on the admission service as attendings and supervisors at Dorothea Dix

Hospital were advanced candidates in the Psychoanalytic Institute, and 65% of the staff at the hospital were now board certified.

The program now stands as a model for other programs in North Carolina and perhaps other states. Nearby Duke University has embarked on a similar venture with John Umstead Hospital, a sister state hospital in the north central region. East Carolina University is in the planning stage for a similar merger with Cherry Hospital in the eastern region and Bowman Gray Department of Psychiatry is negotiating with Broughton Hospital in the western region. At least for North Carolina, this system seems to be enhancing and broadening the residency education experience and, more importantly, has improved recruitment and retention to the state. We have solid evidence that our graduates not only join the university department of psychiatry but also are retained within the state system, in state hospitals, and in community mental health centers where they are so badly needed.

STATE-UNIVERSITY COLLABORATION:
THE UTAH EXPERIENCE

David A. Tomb, M.D.

Leonard J. Schmidt, M.D.

Bernard I. Grosser, M.D.

In many respects, the state-university mental health relationship in Utah reflects the results of a natural experiment. With slightly more than one million people, Utah is a sparsely populated state, a state in which the majority of the professionals either know each other personally or know of one another. Utah has one medical school, one department of psychiatry, one state hospital, one division of mental health, and only three significant population centers, each one a mere fifty miles from its neighbor. Moreover, there is a relatively homogeneous, well-educated population, 80% of which is concentrated in the three cities, while the remaining 20% is spread evenly throughout the vast reaches of this arid, mountainous state. There are no slums, no ghettos, little real poverty, little crime, and, until 20 years ago, no public mental health system outside of a single state hospital.

Thus, Utah can be thought of as an experiment in nature: a state with a well-established department of psychiatry containing a number of professionals well-known in the community, which attempted to develop over a short period of time, a public mental health system from scratch. Given such ideal beginnings and a tabula rasa, how did we fare?

Early Days: The Promise

Models of mental health care existed in Utah twenty years ago primarily in the form of the private practice of a few psychiatrists; several small psychiatric inpatient units of which one was associated with the University; a state training school for the mentally retarded, and a 1000-bed state hospital. In addition, individual faculty members of the Department of Psychiatry of the University of Utah School of Medicine independently had established small clinics in several rural areas. Then, in the mid 1960's, came the appearance of federal dollars and a desire from many quarters to establish a comprehensive community mental health system.

Facing such an opportunity replete with federal money and unencumbered by a past, the state first turned to the department of psychiatry, the state hospital physicians, and the private pychiatric community for assistance. A psychiatrist was appointed director of the State Division of Mental Health and charged with the development of a state-wide mental health network. The chairman of the department of psychiatry and those faculty members with experience establishing community clinics were asked to help. That moment in the mid 60's represented the high-water mark in the involvement of both psychiatry and the department of psychiatry in the development and direction of the public mental health system at a state level.

Why? What went wrong (if, in fact, it can be said that anything went wrong)?

Early Days: The Problems

The federal dollars and the federal program quickly became a political football. The initial tabula rasa soon became filled in with requirements to be met and procedures to be followed. Constraints on salary, flexibility, and personal clinical practice made the State Director of Mental Health position unattractive to available psychiatrists, causing it to be vacated and then filled by a non-psychiatrist. Moreover, the leadership position clearly required skills and interests other than, divorced from, and even incompatible with the clinical abilities of most available psychiatrists. Political, bureaucratic, and administrative skills became the most highly valued (and, perhaps legitimately, the most useful), and the duties of these individuals became primarily political and administrative.

With the change in state leadership and attitude toward personnel who were neither academic nor clinical, came a mutual disenchantment between the state and academic systems. The state leaders appeared to pursue a course guided by and limited to administrative fidelity to federal guidelines, to the mere management of funds. They did not seek nor seem to want clinical, at least not psychiatric, input. On the other hand, the department of psychiatry found that its clinical expertise was not valued on a state level, either on a program development or a case-by-case basis, and thus redirected its community service energies to helping establish individual, county-based, community mental health centers.

By the early 1970's, little remained of state-university collaboration. Although the university's departments of psychology and social work fared no better, the department of psychiatry was definitely "on the outs" with respect to participation in the mental health system on a state level. Explanations for this unfortunate state of affairs varied, but seemed to center upon the markedly different perceptions in the two camps about the important factors needed to establish a state-wide comprehensive community mental health center system.

However, throughout these years, and even preceding them, an ongoing relationship existed between the department of psychiatry and the Utah State Hospital. The hospital had been a minor but regular training site for psychiatric residents, while graduates of the university's program frequently began their practice by taking a position on the staff of the state hospital. This mutually beneficial arrangement remained essentially unaltered throughout the turbulent years of changing state-university priorities and relationships. In fact, it continues to do so to the present day.

State-University Collaboration: The Intervening Years

Little has changed in the years since the early 70's. In spite of occasional overtures on both sides, no meaningful collaborative or even consultative relationship has developed. This non-relationship has continued in spite of occasional changes in leadership on both sides.

From the state, there seems to continue to be a genuine lack of appreciation of the value of local psychiatric/academic input. If additional expertise is sought, the State Division of Mental Health generally turns to personnel from other divisions within the State Department of Social Services, to professionals from the state hospital or other similar state-run facilities, or to experts from out of state. The occasional state/private/academic committees established over the years to address either policy or clinical issues have quickly died due generally to lack of real interest in their activities or response to their decisions. The exception is the State Board of Mental Health, a committee created by law, which has always had at least one psychiatric participant - currently an associate professor from the department of psychiatry. However, until recently the State Board has generally functioned as an overseeing body, leaving the task of crafting mental health policy to the Division of Mental Health.

From the university, there has been little continued effort to create an enhanced state-university dialogue.

Feeling rebuffed and undervalued, the department of psychiatry has looked elsewhere for locations to apply its community psychiatric expertise. Whether the assumed resistance on the part of the state to psychiatric/academic contributions could ultimately be overcome through persistence has never been tested, and yet history would argue against it without such efforts being preceded by a shift in paradigm by one or both of the sides.

Thus, after twenty years of crossing paths, both the Department of Psychiatry of the University of Utah and the Division of Mental Health of the State of Utah continue to be invested in the provision of mental health care in public settings and do so independently of each other.

Overlapping Interests: The Intervening Years

Although the Department of Psychiatry has not collaborated in any meaningful way with the state agency concerned with the care of the mentally ill, it nevertheless has developed numerous activities in the public sector. Faculty members have participated with the various counties in developing and staffing county mental health centers. These have been settings for resident training as well as common sites of first employment after finishing training. Efforts, although only partly successful, have been made to integrate the psychiatric staff at the Utah State Hospital with the psychiatric faculty at the university. Regular meetings, at the university's behest, have been established among key clinical leaders in the public system. The faculty of the department of psychiatry has taken a leading role over the last several years in revising the state's commitment law. Finally, various faculty members have, from time to time, served on or helped create local or state-wide committees critical to the evaluation and provision of quality mental health care.

All of this self-initiated activity on the part of the Department of Psychiatry has occurred without the help, and at times without the knowledge, of the Division of Mental Health. One is reminded of a pair of oxen pulling the same plow but fighting the yoke that binds them.

A brief review of the ways a department of psychiatry has found to be useful to public psychiatry without the support of its state's mental health agency might be instructive.

The University's Role In Creating Mental Health Centers

In 1965, the chairman of the department of psychiatry chaired the committee which developed the state plan organizing the creation of the community mental health centers. Part of that effort detailed the roles of the Utah State Hospital and the Division of Mental Health in relation to the centers. The chairman was essential to this process primarily because the only professional expertise within the state in setting up such focused mental health clinics lay with department faculty.

Over the preceding several years, two faculty members had established clinics in two rural communities, providing the majority of the professional time in each through regular visits. These professionals saw patients, organized a broader network of care within the local community, and trained paraprofessionals to help with that care, particularly during times when the professionals were not available. In so doing, these faculty members developed a model of psychiatric care in very small, very rural settings that later was used profitably when more formal, county sponsored clinics were established. Just as important was a complex of personal contacts linking the department of psychiatry with these rural communities which exists to this day.

Community Mental Health Centers: Formal Collaboration

Although the State Division of Mental Health personnel were charged with implementing the creation of the mental health centers, their experience was limited. They identified locations and hired staff, but the initial clinical course of these centers was rocky. ¬y the early 1970's, the department chairman was approached by community board members to assist in the search for clinical leadership for the state's most urban catchment area. A former resident, then on the faculty of another medical school, was recruited to write the federal staffing grant and plan and direct the clinical program. The Division of Mental Health provided partial funding during the transitional period.

However, since the centers continued to perceive a need for more expert clinical direction, those in the Salt Lake City area sought out formal relationships with the department of psychiatry. This frequently consisted of regular clinical consultation time, time spent by faculty members in planning programs, direct patient care provided by faculty, and, gradually, the development of psychiatric resident training programs in selected mental health centers.

Although the centers with the oldest formal relationship with the department of psychiatry are those within Salt Lake City, the department has played an equally supportive, although slightly different role in the development of three rural mental health centers. What ultimately became the Bear River Community Mental Health Center, ninety miles from Salt Lake City in Logan, Utah, developed around the rural placement of an advanced resident in psychiatry. He spent the last part of his training in that setting, was heavily supervised by department faculty, and used part of his time working with county officials to create the administrative structure for the center. After he finished his training, he continued (and continues today) his association with that center. A second rural mental health center was established around the nidus of a psychiatric resident who was working as a conscientious objector in Moab, Utah, 350 miles from Salt Lake City. He continued his relationship off and on throughout and after his training, the final result being the establishment of the Moab Community Mental Health Center. Later, another resident provided psychiatric coverage to that out-of-the-way center during his training and three years afterwards. Finally, a third center was begun by a faculty member 150 miles from Salt Lake City in Delta, Utah. It was operated as a psychiatric clinic for several years until transformed by a federal grant into a community mental health center, at which time the connection with the department of psychiatry was discontinued. None of these centers would have been able to open in timely fashion without their close relationship with the department of psychiatry.

Beyond such arrangements with outpatient clinics, the department of psychiatry has provided another clinical service for those centers within Salt Lake City: providing the majority of their psychiatric inpatient care. For more than a decade, the department of psychiatry has maintained a contract with the local mental health centers such that the University Hospital acts as their inpatient service. Initial efforts by the centers to provide such care by themselves fared poorly, leaving their only alternative, placement of their patients at the Utah State Hospital. The university stepped into this breach, to the apparent satisfaction of all, since the relationship continues to this day.

Nonetheless, the State Division of Mental Health played almost no role in developing these relationships, even though its initial charge had been to oversee the creation of the comprehensive mental health system in all its parts. Rather, these links resulted from the meshing of the clinical needs of the developing centers with the available clinical expertise of the department of psychiatry, all seen against a background of personal familiarity and respect between the center directors and department faculty. In retrospect, this course of development seems natural in light of the small size of the professional community and the limited clinical resources available.

The State Hospital and the Department of Psychiatry

Probably the only area of significant collaboration between the state and the university has been in the proper staffing and provision of clinical care at the Utah State Hospital. In large part, this has been a marriage of necessity.

The hospital has long been understaffed. The state has never been successful for long at keeping a full, qualified, and satisfied psychiatric staff through application of its normal personnel policies and procedures. Thus, the Division of Mental Health, which is responsible for the functioning of the state hospital, has relied intermittently upon the department of psychiatry to attract regular psychiatric staff to the hospital and to "plug" temporary gaps with psychiatric residents.

Because such a hit and miss system did not meet the long-term needs of the state hospital and was certainly unsatisfactory to the department of psychiatry, several years ago an alternative and potentially more stable approach was tried. A regular faculty member became the clinical director of the Utah State Hospital. With state and university approval, he attempted to recruit psychiatric staff to the hospital who would also be full-time, tenure track faculty members in the department of psychiatry. Although initially attracting some interest, the experiment was short-lived when it became evident that, even with clinical director support, the new staff-faculty would encounter a crushing patient load and have little time free for research or other academic pursuits. Thus, those new hospital psychiatrists, including the clinical director, who were attracted to the university banner have since drifted into private practice or remain on the university faculty in some other setting.

The core discontinuity that seemed to sabotage this particular experiment was a difference in perspective between the state and the university. The state restricted the legitimate activities of psychiatric professionals exclusively to the provision of clinical care. Not only were research or other academic interests unsupported financially or with time, but faculty members capable of obtaining outside funding for their research efforts would find themselves penalized through loss of benefits or even their jobs if they couldn't cover their clinical bases as well. The university, on the other hand, viewed the state hospital as a potential site for psychiatric research and resident training. It wanted to fill the staff-faculty ranks with individuals whose major commitment was toward scholastic pursuits, with clinical activities occupying only part of their time.

At the time of the inception of this state–university staffing plan the state clearly heard the siren song of a state hospital psychiatric staff filled with high quality professionals. Likewise, the university heard the creation of a major new base for clinical research. So compelling were these songs that both sides were blinded to how disparate, and even incompatible, were their respective perceptions of what a psychiatrist actually should do in a state hospital. The plan failed, leaving a bad taste in several mouths.

Regular Meetings Among Key Community Clinicians

Recognizing how intertwined the university and public systems had become, the chairman of the department of psychiatry took the lead in establishing monthly meetings among the leaders from the various parts of the system. Thus, the chairman of the department of psychiatry, the chief of psychiatric services at the Salt Lake Veterans Administration Hospital, the administrative and the clinical directors of the Salt Lake County Community Mental Health System, the director of the university psychiatric inpatient unit, and the clinical director of the Utah State Hospital all meet regularly.

The foci of these meetings are both administrative and clinical. Notably absent is the director of the Division of Mental Health who allows the administrative director of the County Mental Health System to act in his stead. Not only do these meetings serve as a focal point for the development of future public-university collaboration, but at times they address other levels of public mental health planning.

The University and the Mental Health Law

Over the last five years several key faculty members in the department of psychiatry have been instrumental in effecting changes in the state's civil commitment statute and the statutes in the criminal codes which pertain to the mentally ill.

University faculty have long been active participants in civil commitment hearings. They have provided input in periodic revisions of the commitment law, a process guided by the State Division of Mental Health. But, when persistent pressure from civil libertarians through the 1970's resulted in a statute that many felt had grown clinically "toothless," department faculty led the effort to revise the law through a year-long effort marked by securing law faculty assistance with concepts and draftsmanship, tough and occasionally bitter negotiations with civil liberties attorneys, and lobbying key legislators and opinion makers, significant redress was achieved. A final non-negotiable sticking point was debated by a department faculty member and the leading civil liberties opponent on the floor of the legislature. The department position prevailed, and a more balanced commitment statute resulted.

Within the last three years, and in the psycholegal turbulence that followed the Hinckley decision, the state legislature asked for a review and modification of Utah's criminal statutes regarding insanity. A committee was created to evaluate and, if necessary, modify the law. Department faculty members played the central role in this effort, with the result that the law was modified from "not guilty by reason of insanity" to a combination of that judgment and the "guilty and mentally ill" form.

In both of these cases, the State Division of Mental Health was drawn into the debate secondarily and then asked to take a leadership role. In both cases, they then requested the department of psychiatry's participation. However, in each instance there were potent political forces (e.g., legislators, legal services) insisting on the department's participation. Whether the psychiatric/legal interface is in an area of natural state-university collaboration remains unproven at this time.

The University and the Public System: Individual Efforts

The department of psychiatry has had an impact on public mental health care not only through departmental efforts but also through the independent activities of its faculty members. These, of course, are many and varied and have been going on in one form or another for many years. A sample of recent individual efforts is illustrative.

An associate professor in the department and the chief of the VA Psychiatry Service is a member of the State Board of Mental Health. This is a three-year appointment made by the governor and allows the university's voice to be heard at the level of state-wide mental health policy.

Several years ago an assistant professor helped found a self-help support group for the families of the chronically mentally ill; a group which has gone on to become the Utah chapter of the National Alliance for the Mentally Ill (NAMI). This faculty member, in addition to participating in support meetings of members and giving public lectures, has served as president and vice-president of that organization. Moreover, the Utah Alliance for the Mentally Ill has developed close but independent ties with all phases of the public mental health system, including the State Division of Mental Health - thus providing, through the back door, a conduit between the state and the university.

An assistant professor has been appointed to the State Media Committee for Mental Health, a group that operates under the aegis of the Division of Mental Health and has as a mission, riding herd on the media to assure that the mentally ill are dealt with fairly and to help destigmatize mental diseases. This faculty placement was apparently made because of personal contacts between this individual and various personnel in the Division and was related to the frequency with which he made presentations before lay audiences.

An instructor in psychiatry has been appointed to the Salt Lake Board of Mental Health, the board that directs mental health policy in Salt Lake City. Again, this appointment was made through personal contacts, rather than through an effort to have university opinion and expertise represented on a public policy-making body.

Lessons Learned

In a small state, personalities count for more than protocol. Although official lines of communication between agencies are important in "getting the job done," equally important are the sub rosa and informal connections that exist between individuals.

The department of psychiatry has had, and continues to have, a major impact in the development and operation of the public mental health system within Utah and particularly within Salt Lake City. This has been primarily on a clinical/educational level, although ramifications of that contribution have been felt at an administrative level as well. This impact has occurred primarily because of the real clinical needs of the public system; needs the department of psychiatry has had the expertise to help satisfy. In the process, of course, the department faculty members have had to "get their hands dirty" by participating on the front lines caring for the most profoundly ill of psychiatric patients. However, in so doing, faculty's position as experts and teachers has been consolidated with further requests for their input and assistance.

Thus, the department of psychiatry has made its mark on public mental health in Utah by providing clinical expertise in the care of the sickest of patients; expertise unavailable elsewhere. Unfortunately, this contribution generally has been without the support or recognition of the State Division of Mental Health. The state's concerns have been more administrative and programmatic and have seemed to carry the implicit assumption that the nuts and bolts clinical issues were of secondary importance and would get resolved somehow.

Not surprisingly, the focus of the mental health center staffs, directors of the various clinical programs, and concerned families was in line with that of the department of psychiatry and distinctly different from the primary interests of the leaders in the state. Although the Division of Mental Health had different concerns and priorities, and remained uninterested in eliciting a contribution from the department of psychiatry, this stance hasn't mattered. The department has had its impact without such support.

Unfortunately, the loss is in what might have been. No funds have been made available from the State Division for research or training through the department of psychiatry, even at a clinical level and addressing exclusively clinical problems. Nor have the department faculty been used for the training of other personnel, either within the division or throughout the state. At times this approach has produced a manufactured inefficiency, such as when experts have been imported to provide training already available within the department of psychiatry.

The reasons for the continued isolation of the state from the university are not clear. The separation is partly a matter of pressures and priorities, since the one system must respond first to political realities, while the other responds primarily to clinical ones. The separation is also paradigmatic: individuals elect to work in one system or the other, in part, because their world view identifies the system's variables as the important ones. However, some of the continuing division also seems to be associated with issues like turf dispute, wariness of a potential rival, competitiveness, and a determination to avoid the situation of 25 years ago when the psychiatric "establishment" had a lock on mental health care.

So, Utah's "experiment in nature" suggests that good will and a clean slate are not enough. Some sharing of problems, pressures, priorities, paradigms, and even personnel may be essential before systems as disparate as those of the state and the university collaborate meaningfully. And yet, we in Utah continue to hope for that collaboration, since we know how far we have come without it and can imagine our progress if only it had been present.

STATE AND UNIVERSITY COLLABORATION IN THE PROVISION OF PSYCHIATRIC CARE: THE PENNSYLVANIA PERSPECTIVE

Scott Nelson, M.D.

Pennsylvania's public mental health system is the fourth largest in the United States. Its overall budget exceeds $600 million, and over 13,000 persons are employed in the 16 state mental hospitals, half of which are located in urban areas and half in rural settings. The community mental health program provides $125 million to counties which contract with mental health providers for an array of mental health services. The counties receive about $100 million of state funds supplemented by $25 million of Federal Block Grant and Title XX Funds. Monies are allocated by the State Mental Health Authority through a sophisticated performance and need-based process. The community mental health program in Pennsylvania also is responsible for the licensing of private mental health service programs.

Seven university-based departments of psychiatry provide training in Pennsylvania. Five are located in Philadelphia (Hahnemann, Jefferson, Medical College of Pennsylvania, Temple, and the University of Pennsylvania). The remaining two are part of the University of Pittsburgh and Hershey Medical Center. The seven departments graduate approximately 70 residents per year.

Because of concerns expressed about the number and quality of psychiatrists in the state mental hospital system, a survey of psychiatric manpower was conducted by the Pennsylvania State Office of Mental Health in 1980. The survey demonstrated that while there were many dedicated and competent psychiatrists on state mental hospital staff, both quantity and quality of psychiatrists working in the state mental hospital system could be improved substantially. The survey pointed out that the average salary of a staff psychiatrist in a state mental hospital in Pennsylvania was $38,500, the third lowest in the nation. As a result, in 1981, the governor negotiated with the physicians' union a new four-year contract which upgraded the base physician salaries, established a $5,000 board certification bonus (up from $1,000), established a $2,000 per year retention payment which would be paid after each full year of service, and established a performance-based bonus payment which increased from $1,000 to $5,000 per year over five years. In 1983, an additional supplemental bonus package was approved for the state forensic hospital which has encountered special problems in recruitment and retention of psychiatrists.

These increases in monetary rewards have led to improvement in both number and quality of psychiatrists working in state mental health programs, as well as in community mental health programs (whose state funding participation in psychiatrist salaries depends on the state salary and bonus levels). However, it is clear that the amount of money earned by psychiatrists was not the only, nor necessarily even the most important element to success in recruitment and retention of psychiatrists in the public sector. Rather, non-monetary incentives, such as affiliations with medical school departments of psychiatry and other teaching facilities, improved state mental hospital work environments, provision of interesting clinical assignments, and rewards for physicians to take on leadership positions also needed to be provided.

Implementing these incentives has provided significant challenges. Many of the state mental hospitals in Pennsylvania are geographically remote from urban settings and schools of medicine. State mental hospital buildings are often antiquated; many public patients are chronic and difficult to treat, and the state hospital setting continues to suffer from a largely undeserved reputation as an unpleasant setting in which to work. In addition, government personnel rules and regulations pose contraints on the kinds of incentives which can be offered. Some departments of psychiatry do not wish to focus on chronic mentally ill patients, and others show little interest in collaboration with the state.

In spite of theses challenges, however, major strides have been made in the relationship between the state mental health program and university departments of psychiatry in Pennsylvania. Since the late 1970's the Department of Psychiatry at the University of Pittsburgh, lead by Thomas Detre, M.D., has made a major commitment to public service. All full-time faculty must spend three hours per week in service to public mental health programs. Such service has included training and education of community and state hospital mental health providers, technical assistance to state and local programs in which residents receive a salary supplement during their residency in return for a promise to work in a Pittsburgh area state mental hospital after graduation. While there is no direct fiscal or administrative relationship between the state and the department of psychiatry, the state, for its part, provides support for the department's $6.2 million state budget allocation and has lent support to the department's application for federal grants, many of which have been highly successful.

The Commonwealth operated the Eastern Pennsylvania Psychiatric Institute (EPPI), a research and training oriented mental health institute, for 20 years after it was opened in 1959. In 1980, the Department determined that it could no longer operate the Institute, and a serious question was raised as to whether the Institute should be closed. After much debate, the decision was made to determine the interest of medical schools in operating the Institute; the Medical College of Pennsylvania (MCP), developed the best proposal to do so. The Institute is now operated under contract between the state and MCP which has fully integrated its research and training operation into the facility. One of the successfully-met major challenges in the transfer to medical school operation was to accommodate the concerns of employee unions. MCP through EPPI now provides training and education for state mental hospital and community mental health providers in the eastern half of Pennsylvania. In addition, through new publicly oriented department faculty, relationships have been established between MCP and both Haverford State Hospital and Eastern State School and Hospital (the state children's psychiatric hospital).

Direct contracts between departments of psychiatry and state mental hospitals also have been negotiated to provide training and service of mutual benefit. For example, the department of psychiatry at Hahnemann provides the psychiatric coverage for two units including the forensic ward, at Philadelphia State Hospital, as well as on-call coverage on evenings and weekends via contract. Similarly, Hahnemann has a contract to operate the prison mental health program for the city of Philadelphia. A forensic fellowship program is being established between Hahnemann and the state. Similar but smaller contracts have also been effected with the departments of psychiatry at Hershey and Jefferson.

The primary factor in the success of state and university collaborative efforts, in Pennsylvania's experience, has been the presence of individuals on both sides who are committed to public mental health programs, who have an open attitude towards collaboration and the solution of problems, and who are willing to move past parochial concerns to achieve common goals. The development of mutually compatible goals is frequently a major barrier to successful state/university collaboration.

State mental health agencies are primarily responsible for delivery of state mental health services, directly through state mental hospitals, and directly or indirectly through community mental health programs. Departments of psychiatry are concerned with providing opportunities for research and relevant training experiences for residents. Finding areas where these goals can overlap requires persistence, openness, and plain hard work. Without commitment on both sides, the chances of success are minimal.

In summary, successful collaborations between state mental health agencies and university-based departments of psychiatry in Pennsylvania involve the following necessary ingredients:

1. A commitment to finding and achieving goals and objectives, the achievement of which will lead to mutual benefits;

2. An attitude of openness in which solutions to problems are more important than concerns about turf;

3. A mutual positive orientation towards the public mental health system and seriously mentally ill patients;

4. Recognition of the realities in which state mental health agencies and universities operate, i.e., the constraints, rules and regulations, laws, and operating philosophies of each party;

5. A commitment to high quality of effort and results.

While some models are touted as solutions to state/university collaboration, it is our belief that such collaborations need to be tailored in accordance with the individuals in key leadership positions and with the realities of the state and university departments involved. To the extent that those who attempt such collaborations can keep the important factors for success in mind, the public mental health system, the university, and the seriously mentally ill will benefit.

UNIVERSITY AND STATE COOPERATION IN PSYCHIATRIC EDUCATION:

THE ROCHESTER EXPERIENCE

Haroutun M. Babigian, M.D.

Anthony F. Lehman, M.D., M.S.P.H.

In this chapter, we describe the establishment of an innovative joint venture in psychiatric education between the Department of Psychiatry of the University of Rochester School of Medicine and Dentistry and the Rochester Psychiatric Center of the New York State Office of Mental Health. The new program integrates a curriculum on chronic mental disorders and public psychiatry into an existing general psychiatric residency training program. This program illustrates how creative relationships can be developed in the 1980's between academic departments of psychiatry and state public mental health institutions. We also discuss issues that both state and academic institutions need to address and resolve to ensure mutually rewarding relationships.

Historical Context

The location and content of medical graduate education programs reflect the prevailing attitudes, practice patterns, and state of the art of the field. Patterns of psychiatric graduate education underwent substantial change following World War II. Prior to World War II, psychiatric training was based in large state and federal institutions. A 1927 report (1) on approved internships and residencies showed training positions at 270 hospitals with a combined capacity of 155,962 beds. Of the 1,699 residency positions reported at that time, 360 (21%) were in neuropsychiatry, offered in 80 hospitals. Other residency positions included: surgery - 249, internal medicine - 200, tuberculosis - 157, pediatric - 133, and obstetrics and gynecology - 105. Of the 80 hospitals offering neuropsychiatry residencies, 50 had over 1,000 beds, and 40 of these (80%) were large federal or state mental institutions. These 40 facilities accounted for 242 (67%) of the 360 neuropsychiatry residency positions.

After World War II, two major events changed the face of psychiatry and of psychiatric education. The first was the establishment of the National Institute of Mental Health to promote psychiatric research and education and facilitate the development of psychiatric services. The second was the enactment of the Hill-Burton Act, which provided new federal support for the construction of general hospital beds, thus enhancing development of psychiatric units in community hospitals and university teaching hospitals. These events effectively shifted the emphasis of psychiatric training from large state institutions to university teaching hospitals and general hospitals. A result of this shift was an increased training emphasis on acute psychiatric conditions and a fascination with neurotic disorders. The major psychotic disorders were de-emphasized, and chronic patients were left to be cared for by the large state institutions.

A large number of university and general hospitals developed their own residency training programs despite continuation of many residency programs in state institutions. However, the development of this dual system of service and education did not discourage affiliations between university departments of psychiatry and state institutions. As indicated by a 1980 survey of commissioners and chairmen (2), 76% of respondents reported a current relationship between at least one of their state hospitals and a department of psychiatry, and 60% indicated that the relationship was used for training of university residents. However, only 15% of the respondents reported integrated residency programs. According to this survey, the most important factors for insuring good state hospital educational experiences include varied patient populations and clinical experiences, coupled with quality teaching and supervision. The most important product of the state hospital experience is residents' access to a wider variety of patients and services, and exposure to administration and public psychiatry. Major drawbacks in using state hospitals for residency education settings are geographic distance and potentially poor teaching and supervision. Notable successes in integrating university and state training programs have been described in Maryland and Oregon (3, 4).

Local Context

The Monroe County Insane Asylum was established in 1864. With the creation of the New York State Department of Mental Hygiene in 1891, the state assumed responsibility for operation of the asylum, and the Rochester State Hospital was established, now known as the Rochester Psychiatric Center (RPC). Originally, the state hospital was located outside the city, distant from populated areas. As the suburbs grew, the location of the Rochester State Hospital became central in the county. Fortuitously, the medical school and the university hospital

were built within a mile of the state hospital. The muni-
cipal hospital was attached to the university hospital and
contained a 16-bed psychiatric unit. At that time, psychiatry was a division of the university's department of
medicine.

In 1946, under the leadership of Dr. John Romano,
the department of psychiatry was established as a major
department within the School of Medicine and Dentistry.
While the Rochester Psychiatric Center continued its own
residency program until 1982, the department of psychiatry developed a major psychiatric residency training
program separate from that of the state institution.

Relations between the department of psychiatry and
the state hospital were always cordial, with department
faculty providing some consultation at the state facility,
and some state institution psychiatrists joining the university clinical faculty. In the late 1950's and early 1960's,
psychiatric residents from the University of Rochester
rotated for three months at the state hospital. The
rotation was a general one, without the benefit of full-
time faculty supervision. Residents were placed on any of
the hospital's large units, carried very large caseloads
(typically 200-300 patients), and received no specific
teaching about chronic mental disorders or public psychiatry. For example, one of us (HMB) began psychiatric
residency training in July, and was assigned to the state
hospital in September for three months, assuming responsibility for an entire building with approximately 300 female
patient. It so happened that the unit director and the state
hospital resident were on vacation at that time. The state
hospital staff, including the hospital director made a
valiant attempt to provide supervision and teaching which
were extremely valuable, but as is often the case in the
public sector, this was an added responsibility on top of an
already overextended workload. These, and a variety of
other problems led to the discontinuation of this rotation
in 1963. The Rochester State Hospital residency program
had no formal relationship with the university, other than
the occasional rotation of a selected resident through the
university outpatient programs for a six month period. In
the mid-1970's, the university agreed to provide a didactic
program for state hospital residents, funded by an annual
$10,000 contract through the State Office of Mental
Health. In addition, one senior university faculty member
provided weekly rounds for RPC residents for several

years. This arrangement was not successful in recruiting psychiatrists to work at RPC. During the 36 years between 1946 and 1982, only one resident trained at the university chose to work at the Rochester Psychiatric Center, and then only part-time beginning 15 years after completion of training.

Following two years of negotiation and preparation, a special contract was developed in 1982 between the university and the Rochester Psychiatric Center to add six residents to the university residency, two each in the PGY 2, 3, and 4 years, with the provision that all PGY-2 residents rotate through the Evaluation and Training Unit (ETU) at the state facility. Additionally, the contract provides for two chief residents (PGY-4) to spend six month rotations on that unit. In effect, the state supports the training of six residents added to the university's residency contingent and two additional faculty at the university required for the expansion of the training program.

Within the university department of psychiatry, a major new division was established in 1981 for the study and care of the chronically mentally ill, under the direction of Dr. Anthony Lehman. The Evaluation and Training Unit at the Rochester Psychiatric Center was developed as a component of this division. The division also has responsibility for the extended care clinic at the department of psychiatry, continuing care of a large number of mentally ill boarding home residents, and education of students and residents in public psychiatry and the care of chronically mentally ill. Throughout contract development, it was stressed that a single residency training program would replace the dual system previously maintained. With accreditation and enrollment problems facing the state residency training program, it was hoped that this new arrangement would enhance the prospects of the state facility in recruitment of graduates of the university residency training program. This special residency program was established on July 1, 1982, with a major goal of having several residency graduates working at the Rochester Psychiatric Center within five years.

Factors Related to Program Development

During the 1960's and 1970's, very few residents who trained in residencies outside the state system chose to work in state facilities in spite of competitive salaries. It evolved that foreign medical graduates became the primary candidates for the state residency programs, and many continued to work in the state facilities following residency. Federal restrictions on foreign medical graduates under Public Law 94-484 and a general decline in selection of the psychiatry specialty by medical graduates gradually led to a crisis in psychiatric staffing of the state facilities. To seek solutions to this problem, Dr. James Prevost, then New York State Commissioner of Mental Health, met with a group of chairmen of departments of psychiatry to discuss possible strategies. Training funds were available through the existing state residency training programs, but needed to be channeled in ways that would enhance recruitment and retention of psychiatrists for the centers.

During that time, Dr. Frank Soults, Medical Director at the Rochester Psychiatric Center, favored the establishment of expanded relations with the University of Rochester for a variety of reasons. Not only would university involvement be of potential assistance in resolving recruitment problems, but it would provide access to a wider variety of resources and incentives. Additionally, the university liaison could be a powerful ally in responding to growing political and public pressure to improve the image and quality of care provided at the state facility.

For a somewhat different set of reasons, Dr. Haroutun Babigian, Chairman of the Department of Psychiatry of the University of Rochester School of Medicine and Dentistry, favored development of expanded relations with the state. First, dwindling available funding for training programs forced the department of psychiatry to seek new sources of financial support. Second, the recent shift toward the medical model and study of biological foundations of mental illness led to renewed interest in understanding and care of chronic mental illness and the more severe disorders. The need for well trained psychiatrists to care for the chronically mentally ill in the public sector became apparent with the change of focus. In addition, Dr. Babigian had a strong personal commitment to increased department involvement in public psychiatry and care of the chronically mentally ill.

The following factors were essential to the successful implementation of this cooperative program: 1)   A
clear understanding by all parties (the University, RPC,
and the State Office of Mental Health) that, in order to
enhance recruitment of university-trained psychiatrists by
the state facility, a joint integrated program was needed
which emphasized study and care of the chronically
mentally ill and taught principles and issues of public
psychiatry. 2)   The university department of psychiatry,
through faculty recruitment and curriculum emphasis, had
to make a significant commitment to the study and care of
the chronically mentally ill and to the teaching of public
psychiatry. This was accomplished through the creation of
a special division within the department. 3) Under supervision of full-time faculty from the university, residents
needed to rotate through a special unit at the state institution, focusing on the evaluation and treatment of the
most difficult chronically mentally ill patients in that
institution.   4)   Residents had to be able to come to an
understanding that work with the chronically mentally ill
patient can be rewarding, and that major breakthroughs in
psychiatry are dependent upon careful evaluation and
treatment of these patients.   5)   The state needed to
understand that it must support education of residents in a
special way not solely dependent upon inpatient training.
With the addition of six residents to the existing university
program, all residents were able to rotate through the
state institution.   The state residency training contract
also paid for support of the training of residents at the
university.   The state agreed that training at the state
facility would be concentrated in a 50-bed unit, and not
dispersed throughout the entire institution of approximately 900 beds. 6) The university had to commit itself
to place excellent faculty at the RPC unit, and to assume
responsibility for the continued nurturance and development of that faculty.   7)   The university assumed total
responsibility for recruitment and selection of residents
and development of curriculum.

Program Goals

The basic goals of the residency training contract between the State Office of Mental Health and the university department of psychiatry were as follows:

1. To expand the department of psychiatry's curriculum in chronic care and public psychiatry;

2. To improve the quality of care at the Rochester Psychiatric Center;

3. To develop clinical and training modalities applicable to other state-operated facilities;

4. To enhance the recruitment and retention of clinical staff, particularly psychiatrists, at RPC;

5. To develop research programs on the nature and treatment of chronic mental disorders.

Description of the New Residency Training Unit

A major focus and innovation of the contract was the creation of a jointly operated 50-bed residency training unit at the Rochester Psychiatric Center known as the Evaluation and Training Unit. While many joint programs between state and university are created with a partial goal of increasing university access to beds, this was not a factor in the development of the ETU. The department of psychiatry already had 107 beds, and these were not fully staffed by residents, so there was no need to develop additional training sites for this reason. Rather, the university's primary goal in this joint effort was expansion of curriculum. The purposes of this unit are:

1. Clinical assessment and treatment of chronically mentally disabled young adults between the ages of 18 and 35;

2. Training of psychiatric residents, medical students, and other professional mental health trainees in the care of chronic mental patients;

3.   Provision of continuing education for other RPC staff;

4.   Development of research on the nature and treatment of chronic mental disorders.

This unit selected the young adult population with severe chronic mental disorders because of the rising numbers of "young chronic patients" in the public mental health system, and concerns regarding the increasing pressures these patients place on inpatient services.

The Unit and Staffing

The Evaluation and Training Unit consists of two 25-bed wards, including an assessment ward and a rehabilitation ward.   The assessment ward focuses on indepth clinical assessment of the biological, psychological, and social problems and strengths of patients. During an 8-10 week evaluation period, several standardized clinical assessments are completed, focusing on diagnosis, response to past psychiatric treatment, family relations, social network, and practical skills needed to cope with life outside the hospital.   On the basis of this extensive evaluation, a treatment plan is developed for the patient. The ward provides various kinds of treatment for these patients, including medication trials, behavior modification programs, family counseling, and social skills training. The rehabilitation ward, opened in October, 1984, complements this process by providing an extended, behaviorally oriented, skill-building inpatient program to prepare difficult-to-place young adult chronic patients for community living.
The ETU is jointly staffed by the University of Rochester and the Rochester Psychiatric Center, with most of the clinical staff coming from RPC. The unit chief is jointly employed by RPC and the university, and has full academic faculty appointment. Other key clinical personnel, including other psychiatrists, psychologists, and a social worker and nurse are full time university faculty. With the exception of two staff development faculty and a computer programmer hired through the university, other staff are employees of the Rochester Psychiatric Center.

Training on the Evaluation and Training Unit

Consistent with the model of a jointly operated residency training program, all university psychiatric residents rotate through the training unit at the Rochester Psychiatric Center. Under this model, all PGY-2 residents spend three months on the unit as team physicians and primary therapist for patients. At a given time, each resident carries 5-6 patients as primary therapist and 2-3 patients as medical consultant. Their work is supervised by faculty attending psychiatrists as well as by a PGY-4 chief resident. The resident is expected to perform all the required functions of a physician in a state hospital. During assignment to the ETU, residents also take night call once each week at the RPC. A copy of the residency training curriculum is presented in an appendix to this chapter.

Although the focus of training is on residents, a variety of other professional trainees avail themselves of this program. During their third year clerkship, some medical students spend six-week rotations on the ETU. This clerkship is similar to other clerkships on university wards, with the student assuming primary responsibility for patients under the supervision of residents and faculty. This inpatient experience is supplemented by rounds on acute wards at the university and by emergency room call. Various types of training experiences are also provided for first and second year medical students, graduate nursing students, and occupational and recreational therapy students.

Clinical Program on the Evaluation and Training Unit

Patients are accepted on referral basis from other inpatient programs within the RPC. The criteria for screening include: 1) patient age between 18 and 35 years, 2) diagnosis of a chronic mental disorder of at least two year's duration, and 3) identification of specific evaluation questions related to the patient's clinical care. Very few patients who are referred on the basis of these criteria are excluded from the program. In particular, every effort has been made to avoid "skimming" of easy-to-treat patients from other units, a practice for which university-affiliated programs at state institutions have frequently been criticized.

Once patients arrive on the unit, they undergo an initial clinical evaluation by the treatment team. This evaluation focuses on the identification of acute problems in need of immediate attention, and formulation of treatment problems and goals for the duration of the assessment period. At the end of the first week, a formulation meeting is held with the treatment team, at which the primary therapist presents the case and summarizes the initial problem list and the initial assessment and treatment plans. The patient then undergoes standardized assessments and observation within the subsequent 6-8 weeks; the results of the standardized assessments are reviewed; and revised treatment plans with recommendations for long term care are developed. At this point, patients may be discharged, returned to their home inpatient unit at RPC, or continued on the Evaluation and Training Unit for further rehabilitation and eventual discharge.

Patient Characteristics and Outcomes

As of September, 1984, a total of 105 patients had been evaluated in the evaluation ward of ETU. The demographic and clinical characteristics of these patients are displayed in Tables 1 and 2. Demographically, these patients are similar to the typical young adult chronic patients seen at the RPC. Their level of social dysfunction is underscored by the fact that only 10% were employed prior to the current admission, and 90% had never been married. The most common diagnoses among these patients included schizophrenia (61%) and chronic affective disorders (14%) (see Table 2). Other diagnoses included severe character disorders, organic brain disorders, and various less common diagnoses such as genetic disorders associated with behavioral problems. ˉatients with primary diagnoses of drug or alcohol abuse are not admitted, although many of the patients have substance abuse as a secondary diagnosis. A quarter of the patients had other disabilities secondary to their mental disorders. About half of these had substance abuse as a secondary disability, but several types of physical disability also were represented. Ninety percent of the patients treated came from other inpatient programs at the RPC, including 66% from other long term inpatient programs and 25% from the acute admission unit. The other 10% were referred from outside hospitals and agencies. Of those treated, the mean current length of stay prior to transfer to the ETU was nearly ten months. On the average, it had been eight years since the patients' first psychiatric hospitalization, indicating the chronicity of their illnesses.

Table 2 also illustrates some of the types of problems for which these patients were referred to the unit and the types of problems addressed in assessment and treatment. The most common referral problems included the assessment of alternative treatments, diagnosis, potential for community placement, vocational level, and family problems. Typically referred patients posed major management problems for their home units. Often the patient was referred becaused the home unit felt it had exhausted its options in providing care. Another common scenario was referral of a patient who the current treatment team felt ought to be able to live outside the hospital, but who needed more intensive treatment which they themselves were unable to provide. The most common problem identified on the basis of assessment on the ETU was major difficulty in maintaining appropriate placement in the community, a problem shared by 80% of ETU patients. This problem was typically associated with the absence of a supportive family, absence of a support network outside the hospital, and prior failures at placement in alternative living situations. Several of the patients had caused major problems in group homes or supervised community residences, such that they were not eligible to return to these settings without clearly demonstrating improvements in behavior. Over half of the patients were noncompliant with their treatment, mainly with medication, but also with follow-through for day treatment programs, vocational rehabilitation, and other kinds of psycho-social interventions. Twenty-nine percent of the patients displayed suicidal ideation while on the ETU, and half of these made some sort of suicide attempt. A quarter of the patients were actively violent on the unit, and 24% engaged in unacceptable forms of sexual behaviors. These types of behavioral problems were the main reasons that these patients remained hospitalized, although many of the patients also showed persistent psychotic symptoms in spite of apparently adequate psychopharmacologic treatment. Of the patients evaluated and treated on the ETU to date, the median length of stay has been three months.

An interesting issue that must be evaluated in the development of this type of unit is its impact on the census of the hospital, and the hospital's ability to discharge difficult-to-place patients. While no follow-up data are yet available for ETU patients, preliminary analyses have been conducted comparing patients who were discharged against those who were returned to other inpatient units. These findings begin to address a question that often gnaws at state psychiatric center staff: "If we just had more staff, what might we be able to do with this patient?" As of September, 1984 a total of 82 patients had been either discharged (72%) or transferred (28%) from the unit. Table 3 reveals some trends in differences between these two groups. Of patients discharged, only 12% had no family contacts, compared to 22% of those returned to inpatient programs. This difference begins to illustrate the importance of support networks outside of the hospital in achieving successful discharge. The patients transferred back to other units also had more hospital admissions and had spent considerably longer time in the hospital. Presumably, a combination of factors, including the extensive amounts of time spent in the hospital, contributed to the breakdown of their support networks outside of the hospital. Being suicidal or posing placement problems were not major distinguishing factors between those discharged and those transferred. Violence and noncompliance, behaviors which are clearly unacceptable to community placement programs, were often related to the patient's psychopathology, particularly psychosis that had been unresponsive to psychopharmacologic intervention.

Problems and Issues

A major problem faced by an innovative program such as that described above is its ability to gain acceptance by the rest of the RPC. The ETU has had its difficulties in this regard, although considerable progress has been made in the first two years of its existence. The major issues raised by the creation of such a unit are: 1) perceived intrusion of outsiders, i.e., university personnel, into the fabric of the state facility; 2) the focus of resources on this unit to some extent at the expense of other units; and 3) difficulties in integrating two bureaucracies, i.e., that of the state and the university, to support a clinical program.

Actions that have been taken to alleviate some of these potential conflict areas include: 1) focus of treatment on difficult patients, thus providing some tangible alleviation of clinical problems for other units; 2) development of working liaison relationships with other units to facilitate transfer and removal of patients; 3) provision of additional educational services such as case conferences for staff on other units; 4) participation of unit employees in various functional capacities throughout the institution, such as committee; and 5) regular meetings between the chairman of the department of psychiatry and the executive and medical directors of RPC.

Another problem has been establishing a sense of integration within the department of psychiatry for faculty working at RPC. For these faculty, feeling isolated from the rest of the department can lead to frustration and burn-out. To cope with this problem, these faculty attend regular department grand rounds, maintain office space at the university, collaborate with other faculty on teaching and research projects, and supervise residents in clinical setting besides RPC. Also, faculty based elsewhere in the department act as case consultants on a regular basis on the ETU.

Major Achievements of the Residency Training Contract

Four major achievements resulting from the contract are noteworthy:

1. Despite considerable obstacles against opening the unit, including a reduction in force at the time the unit was scheduled to open and a major change in hospital administration, the unit has opened and has proceeded in its development along the proposed lines.

2. Although the assessment ward itself was not expected to discharge many patients, it has been able to discharge the large majority of those patients evaluated and treated, an achievement much appreciated by the Rochester Psychiatric Center and extremely important in the training of residents to dispel the notion that these patients are untreatable and therefore, unrewarding.

3. Although development of clinical and training programs has to precede the development of research, the unit has received a three-year grant to study the effectiveness of two different types of family management in treatement of schizophrenia, and is participating in a double-blind drug trial of a new antipsychotic medication. These two studies have stimulated a sense of inquiry among unit staff, and a variety of smaller studies of interest to staff are in progress.

4. Although the goal of the program was to recruit one new psychiatrist each year for the RPC, five of seven graduating university psychiatrists have been recruited by RPC by the end of the second year, two within the ETU and three in other areas. Current indications are that more graduating residents will choose to work at RPC in the future. In its first two years, the program has achieved more in terms of recruitment than had been achieved in the previous thirty years. This achievement in itself has done much to solidify the credibility of the unit and program, and has gained increased acceptance by staff of the RPC.

Beyond University and State

The need for training of professionals for roles in public psychiatry is not limited to the state facilities. If adequate community care of chronically mentally ill patients is to become a reality, training in treatment approaches and service needs must be available throughout a range of community contexts. A comprehensive mental health demonstration project is currently being implemented in the Monroe and Livingston County area which has a special focus to coordinate community care of chronic mental patients. This project has potential for large impact on the state facility and community programs and their relationships and training needs.

Context of the Demonstration Project

Monroe and Livingston County constitute the catchment area of the Rochester Psychiatric Center. Within the area is an assortment of mental health services, including a community mental health center, three other community mental health centers attached to hospitals, a county mental health service, a children's hospital and mental health service, and various agencies specializing in residential and rehabilitative care. The combined 1980 population of the two counties was approximately 750,000. With availability of a full range of mental health services and no large communities nearby, this area is reasonably self-sufficient in provision of mental health care.

Since 1979, planning has been underway for a comprehensive set of community solutions for problems in mental health service delivery. Some of the major problems which prompted community mental health leaders to undertake this effort included: 1) failure of funding to follow chronic patients into the community, leading to lack of appropriate available services and options for care; 2) lack of clear area coordination and planning for mental health services based on accurate information about patients and services; and 3) patterns of funding and reimbursement of services which interfere with effective service delivery to populations in need of services. Parties involved in demonstration planning included directors of community mental health centers and the state facility, representatives of the counties and the state, representatives of other local mental health services, and a variety of consultants and staff.

The Demonstration

After almost five years of planning, the demonstration project plan has been fully developed, and has received approval and funding from the state legislature. Concepts developed for the demonstration received heavy endorsement from the 1984 Governor's Select Commission of Mental Health in New York State. The major components of this plan for an integrated mental health system are as follows:

o   **Integrated Mental Health (IMH):**
    IMH is not-for-profit membership corporation which has primary responsibility for planning and administration for mental health for the area. This responsibility includes community policy development, control of funding, identification of service development needs, coordination with

other service sectors (i.e., alcoholism, social services), and management of data systems. Board members consist of local business leaders selected by respective IMH member agencies (CMHCs, state, county, specialized agencies, and United Way).

o   **Contract Revenues System (CRS):**
In the past, mental health agencies have received public funds through a variety of mechanisms, foremost of which was a deficit financing system. Delayed payments, retroactive cuts, and other problems with this funding mechanism created serious obstacles to agencies' ability to utilize funds effectively. The CRS provides for formulated performance contract funding, through which agencies know their budget in advance and are responsible for providing defined volumes of services. With regular agency funding stabilized through the CRS, agencies are able to undertake development of a more responsive system of care for chronic patients and other patients in the community.

o   **Management Information Systems:**
IMH has developed and is in the process of implementing a complex management information system to support planning and coordination of mental health care in the area. Each participating agency is provided access to a comprehensive data system for its internal management of patient and fiscal information. Standardized information is regularly extracted from these files into a central data file which allows for area-wide summaries of important patient and cost data. This central file is organized longitudinally to follow individual patients across facilities and episodes of care while preserving patient confidentiality.

o   **Capitation Payments System (CPS):**
The CPS focuses on improving care for chronic mentally ill individuals within the community. The program's goals include expansion of available services through start-up funding and pay-

ment for services, provision for assignment of responsibility for care of each eligible patient through a capitation mechanism, and provision for funds to follow patients to cover all approrpriate services. For initial program implementation, patient eligibility is defined in terms of previous utilization of inpatient care at the Rochester Psychiatric Center. Eligible patients are devided into three groups, each having a separate capitation rate and responsibility level. The groups are as follows:

Continuous Patients - These patients consist primarily of individuals who have been hospitalized at RPC almost continuously during the last two years (a minimum of 270 days), though they may have spent periods of time outside the hospital. A contract for care of a continuous patient involves responsibility for total patient care, including residential care or health insurance, but responsibility for coordination and quality control of care resides with the contracting agency.

Intermittent Patients - The intermittent group consists of those patients who have had from 30 to 270 days of RPC hospitalization in the past two years. Most of these patients already have some sort of residential and support networks available in the community, though in many cases these provisions are inadequate to prevent exacerbation of illness. A contract for care of an intermittent patient involves responsibility only for delivery of comprehensive mental health and related rehabilitative services, plus overall management of patient care.

Outpatients - Individuals who are currently outpatients at RPC are also eligible for CPS capitation. Contractual responsibility for these patients includes overall patient management and delivery of ambulatory mental health services.

The community mental health centers may serve as lead agencies in contracting for eligible CPS patients. Other agencies participate in care of CPS patients only to the extent that they are asked to do so. Each agency has in its management information system an inquiry file which allows it to determine whether any new patient is already under contract to another agency, and to make appropriate referrals accordingly.

Implications for Future Training

In the context of the demonstration project, methods of caring for chronic patients in the community will be quite different from techniques currently familiar to mental health professionals in the area. Active case management and outreach activities are required in addition to strategies for network development and family support. New community-wide training programs will be required which incorporate these features if professional staff are to be adequately prepared for this type of approach to mental health care.

As we continue to develop more sophisticated systems to care for the chronically mentally ill in the community, our training programs will accommodate the changes. Some of the directions for change include the following: 1) The state hospital needs to become an excellent small inpatient evaluation and treatment planning facility for the chronically mentally ill and must become integrated into the joint fiscal and program planning of the overall community. 2) We need to define the optimal role and timing of the use of hospitalization in the closely coordinated care of chronically mentally ill individuals. The current tendency to view a need for hospitalization as a failure of the system to care adequately for chronic patients is unrealistic and a major factor contributing to staff burnout. 3) New programming also has to recognize the need to treat chronically mentally ill patients within their psychological and social context, as well as providing the more traditional biological forms of treatment.

Graduate training and research should be considered an integral part of any community program for care of the chronically mentally ill, to provide adequate program staffing and approaches to treatment. Recent trends to cut funding and programming in these areas are dangerously short-sighted and should be remediated promptly.

Acknowledgement

The authors would like to extend a special note of thanks to Sylvia Reed, Ph. D. for her extensive editorial assistance in preparation of this chapter.

REFERENCES

1. Hospitals approved for advanced internships or residencies. JAMA 88:828-834, 1927

2. Faulkner LR, Eaton JS Jr, Rankin RM: Administrative relationships between state hospitals and academic psychiatry departments. Am J Psychiatry 140:898-901, 1983

3. Weintraub W, Harbin HT, Book J, et al: The Maryland plan for recruiting psychiatrists into public service. Am J Psychiatry 141:91-94, 1984

4. Faulkner LR, Eaton JS Jr, Bloom JD, et al: The CMHC as a setting for residency education. Community Ment Health J 18:3-10, 1982

Table 1
Cummulative Characteristics of
Patients Treated on the ETU
(November, 1982 – September, 1984)

N = 105
Ethnicity: Caucasian - 74%
               Black   - 22%
               Other   - 4%

Age: Median = 25 years
Sex: Male   - 66%
Marital Status: Never Married - 90%
Living Situation Prior to Current RPC Admission:
    With Family   -   52%
    Independent   -   20%
    Supervised Community Residence   -   9%
    Other Institution   -   2%
    Other   -   17%
Employment Status Prior to RPC Admission:
    Unemployed –   90.4%
    Sheltered Employment   -   1.9%
    Full-Time Employment   -   4.8%
    Part-Time Employment   -   2.9%

Table 2
Cummulative Clinical Characteristics
of Patients Treated on the ETU
(November, 1982 – September, 1984)

N = 105
Reason for ETU Referral:
    Assessment for Treatment Alternatives   – 52%
    Diagnostic Assessment   – 38%
    Discharge/Placement Assessment   – 41%
    Review of Medications   – 42%
    Vocational Assessments   – 27%
    Family Assessment   – 13%
Frequency of Problems Noted on ETU
(in descending order of frequency):
    Community Placement Problems   – 82%
    Noncompliance with Treatment   – 62%
    Threatening Behavior   – 37%
    Suicidal Ideation   – 29%
    Violent Behavior   – 24%
    Inappropriate Sexual Behavior   – 24%
    Tardive Dyskinesia   – 23%
    Suicide Attempts   – 15%

Diagnosis: Schizophrenia   –   61%
    Major Affective Disorder   –   14%
    Other   –   25%

Current length of stay: Prior to ETU transfer:
    median   = 51 days
    mean   = 246 days
    (range   0-2797 days)
    On ETU: median = 90 days
    mean = 123 days
    (range 10-562 days)

Table 3
Comparison of Patients Discharged
vs
Transferred from the ETU
(November, 1982 – September, 1984)

Variable	Discharged (72%)	Transferred (28%)
N	59	23
% Male	66%	70%
% Caucasian	71%	83%
% Never married	85%	100%
% High school graduate	69%	62%
% Voluntary	56%	61%
% Schizophrenia	59%	78%
% Primary family available	88%	78%
% Suicidal on ETU	27%	35%
% Violent on ETU	17%	43%
% Noncompliant on ETU	58%	74%
% Placement problems in community	78%	91%
Median LOS prior to ETU transfer	15 days	330 days
Mean LOS prior to ETU transfer	168 days	450 days
Median LOS on ETU	70 days	138 days
Mean LOS on ETU	107 days	167 days

APPENDIX

Curriculum in Chronic Care and Public Psychiatry for Psychiatric Residents

Overall Goals

The overall goals of this curriculum are: 1) To train residents in the clinical care of chronically disabled psychiatry patients; 2) To interest residents in providing care to these patients after they complete their training; 3) To acquaint residents with the principles of public psychiatry and related fields of knowledge; and 4) To stimulate some residents to pursue professional careers in the public health care sector.

The proposed curriculum is organized to guide residents toward these goals over the three years of their residency. Early in the residency, emphasis is placed on acquisition of requisite clinical skills. As residents progress and feel more comfortable in their clinical roles, the focus moves to the system level, providing residents with information and experiences in the broader field of public psychiatry.

I.   Post-Graduate Year II

    A.   Chronic Care

        1)   Goals

            a)   Learn to assess chronic patients in inpatient settings. This includes:

                (1)   Ability to collect a clinical data base from patients, significant others, hospital chart, initial observations on the ward, and specialized assessment techniques;

                (2)   Ability to use this data base to formulate DSM-III multiaxial diagnoses; hypotheses about the predisposing, precipitating, and perpetuating factors in the patient's illness; and a problem list with specific treatment goals.

b)   Learn to develop inpatient care plans and discharge plans for patients. These include:

  (1)   Translation of treatment goals into specific treatment interventions;

  (2)   Ability to work with the multi-disciplinary care team in defining treatment plans;

  (3)   Ability to communicate these care plans to the patient, significant others, and other professionals.

c)   Learn to provide direct care to chronic patients in the inpatient setting. This includes:

  (1)   Appropriate use of psychotropic medications;

  (2)   Supportive psychotherapy;

  (3)   Organization of structured, goal-directed ward programs designed to support the patient's reconstruction and preparation for discharge or transfer.

2) Educational Activities

a)   Residents will spend three months during PGY-II on the University-Rochester Psychiatric Center Evaluation and Training Unit. This provides direct, supervised experiences in the assessment, planning, and care for chronic patients.

b)   During PGY-II, residents attend a year-long series of didactic presentations on major psychiatric disorders, neuro-psychiatry, psycho-pharmacology, ECT, and several other areas related to the inpatient care of chronic patients.

B. Public Psychiatry

1) Goals

a) Introduce residents to the public psychiatric hospital.

b) Acquaint residents with the aftercare system in Monroe County available to their inpatients.

2) Educational Activities

a) Inpatient rotation on Evaluation and Training Unit.

II. Post-Graduate Year III

A. Chronic Care

1) Goals

To extend residents' experience with chronic patients beyond the hospital's walls. Specifically:

a) Learn to use psychotropic medications for "maintenance" therapy, including: minimization of dosage, drug holidays, judicious use of antiparkinson agents, recognition and treatment of acute and long-term side effects, particularly tardive dyskinesia.

b) Establish ongoing therapeutic relation-ships with chronic patients and their significant others with an orientation toward education about illness and treatments, identification of assets as well as needs, one-to-one patient-therapist relationship, awareness of counter-transference in the care of chronic patients.

c) Become familiar with the community-based system of care for these patients and how to integrate the psychiatrist's services with these other services, including referrals, consultations, and case management.

2) Educational Activities

a) Act as psychiatric consultants for a group of chronic outpatients in the University's Extended Care Clinic.

b) At least once during the course of the year, do each of the following in connection with the care of a patient: meet in consultation with the staff of a community clinic, provide medical follow-up (e.g., for medication renewal) at a local residential care facility; meet with a patient's family or significant others; visit the County Department of Social Services; visit a sheltered work setting. All of these activities should be enhanced by one-to-one supervision from a faculty member.

c) Participate in the seminar on Clinical Epidemiology, Public Psychiatry, and Long-Term Care.

B. Public Psychiatry

1) Goals

To broaden residents' knowledge base and experiences in public psychiatry. Specifically:

a) To acquaint them with the fields of forensic psychiatry, health care legislation, medical economics, and community psychiatry.

        b)   To give them direct experiences in each of these areas.

    2)   Education Activities

        a)   Residents will participate in the seminar on Clinical Epidemiology, Public Psychiatry, and Long-Term Care.

III.   Post-Graduate Year IV

    A.   Chronic Care

        1)   Goals

To solidify residents' expertise in the psychiatric management of chronic patients and to encourage some to make a major professional commitment to the field of chronic care.

        2)   Educational Activities

            a)   A variety of elective experiences are provided, including:
                (1)   Chief Resident on the Evaluation and Training Unit;

                (2)   Clinical rotation in another inpatient or outpatient unit at Rochester Psychiatric Center;

                (3)   Research project in the field of chronic care.
            Faculty supervision will be provided for all these activities.

            b)   Weekly consultation on patients at the Sociolegal Clinic.

    B.   Public Psychiatry

        1)   Goals

To provide residents with experience in administrative psychiatry and to encourage some to pursue a career in public psychiatry.

2) Educational Activities

    a) Participate in the Administrative Psychiatry seminar. In this seminar, basic systems and organizational theory are presented, and most of the time is devoted to residents' presentations of their administrative experiences to the group in order to develop skills in organizational consultations.

    b) For interested residents, elective experiences are provided with supervision, including:

        (1) Extended experience in forensic psychiatry;

        (2) Research project in mental health care services.

THE GALT VISITING SCHOLAR IN
PUBLIC MENTAL HEALTH:
A VIRGINIA EXPERIENCE

Joseph Bevilacqua, Ph.D.

Background and Rationale

The tumultuous changes that have affected mental health practice and education are paradoxical. I use the word paradoxical purposefully. As we have developed a clearly sophisticated technology in the care and treatment of mental illness and are moving toward a biological-oriented frame of reference in research and education, the public practice sector appears to be increasingly isolated from this development. Furthermore, the attendant fiscal instruments are reinforcing this isolation. And finally, the psycho-social developments in public practice are themselves isolated from the mainstreams of activities in the university and corporate sectors. We have, therefore, very different developments on different tracks - but moving away from a common center. It is this disparity - this persistent two-class system that is the hub of the paradox in the American system of the care of the mentally ill.

The elements of change include the changing role of the federal government in health and human services, emerging mental health constituency, exploding corporate development in psychiatric hospitals, and a shifting financial base for psychiatric education and training. These developments attest to ferment and uncertainty in the future direction for public mental health services.

The increasing visibility of chronic mentally ill people and their relationship to the homeless is only one current expression of concern within the public mental health system in this country. The ravages of the policy of deinstitutionalization, either real or apparent, have been a part of these contemporary developments.

It was with these issues in mind as well as a growing concern about the increasing isolation of the public mental health system from mainstream academic practice that Dr. James Prevost and I first conceived and then developed the Galt Visiting Scholar Program in Virginia.

We purposely chose to honor the name of Galt, because this family provided the initial leadership for the first free-standing public mental hospital in the United States located in Williamsburg, Virginia. From 1773 until the mid-1800's, members of the Galt family served as administrators and physicians to this hospital. The professionalization of care was a major hallmark of this family's contribution to the mentally ill of early America. (1)

The rationale of developing a scholar's focus was deliberate. In Virginia during the late 1970's and early 1980's, the relationship of the state hospitals to the university was inactive and lacked any continuing systemic relationship. They were, in short, two publicly supported systems whose directions and operations touched hardly at all.

In 1982, House Joint Resolution No. 112 was passed by the Virginia General Assembly. It stated:

> RESOLVED by the House of Delegates, the Senate concurring, That state-supported institutions of higher education which train individuals to work in professions associated with mental illness, mental retardation or substance abuse are requested to develop cooperative relationships with the Department of Mental Health and Mental Retardation. The Department and state-supported educational institutions shall strive to improve the capability of the Department of Mental Health and Mental Retardation to recruit qualified professionals to work in state and community mental health, mental retardation, and substance abuse programs.
>
> In addition, the universities and medical schools shall (are requested to) cooperate with the ongoing work of the Department to evaluate staffing requirements for state hospitals and training centers and to determine the appropriate levels of care to be provided by state facilities and community programs for the mentally handicapped. The Department and educational institutions shall seek to foster internships and work experience opportunities for students and staff of the universities and medical schools; and be it
>
> RESOLVED FURTHER, That the Clerk of the House of Delegates is requested to forward a copy of this resolution to each of the state institutions of higher education which train mental health and medical professionals."(2)

An important consideration in forging the resolution's intent was to engage the key leadership of those universities which had medical schools. A formal agreement was developed between the University of Virginia, Virginia Commonwealth University, and the Eastern Virginia Medical Authority. Signatores include the Presidents of the three universities, the Commissioner of the Department of Mental Health and Mental Retardation and the Governor. The funding was to be by the Department of Mental Health and Mental Retardation, and the scholar was to be located in the Universities' Department of Psychiatry and Behavioral Medicine, as a visiting professor.

The agreement states the following:

The Virginia Department of Mental Health and Mental Retardation, and the University of Virginia, Virginia Commonwealth University, and the Eastern Virginia Medical Authority jointly agree to the establishment and support of the Galt Visiting Scholar in Public Mental Health. This will acknowledge and honor the significant contribution of the Galt Family who provided the initial leadership in the creation of the first public psychiatric hospital in the United States, in Williamsburg, Virginia in 1773.

The establishment of the Galt Visiting Scholar in Public Mental Health will be consistent with the intent of House Joint Resolution 112, whereby the Virginia General Assembly in its regular 1982 session identified "the need to strengthen professional ties between State Hospitals and training centers for the mentally handicapped and Virginia universities and medical schools...(and) to develop cooperative relationships with the Department of Mental Health and Mental Retardation."

In order to implement the Galt Visiting Scholar Program in public mental health, a cooperative effort between the Department of Mental Health and Mental Retardation and the University of Virginia, Virginia Commonwealth University and the Eastern Virginia Authority will pertain.

The primary focus of the Visiting Scholar will be to strengthen the professional ties between the Department of Mental Health and Mental Retardation and the University of Virginia, Virginia Commonwealth University and the Eastern Virginia Medical Authority. Attention will be paid to the professional preparation and its application to the public mental health system. The policy implications for mental health care and the necessary support services for the mentally disabled will be a part of the inquiry associated with the Galt Scholar. The perspective will be interdisciplinary with the engagement of all pertinent disciplines and university programs. (3)

The responsibilities of the Galt Scholar were to include the following: (4)

1. Identify and analyze contemporary issues related to current public mental health practices.

2. Assess policies and programs designed to improve treatment and management practices for public mental health services.

3. Establish and maintain clinical relationships with the University of Virginia, Virginia Commonwealth University, and the Eastern Virginia Medical Authority with emphasis on education and training of psychiatrists and other mental health professionals.

4. Assist universities in assessing public mental health practices and procedures so that they may be aware of the needs of the public system.

5. Serve as primary link between the Department of Mental Health and Mental Retardation, the universities and the medical schools in identifying and establishing program relationships with public programs and other health care and psycho-social professionals.

In practice, the Galt Scholar position would minimize bureaucratic concerns with budgets and personnel. The Scholar would be free to move in and between the different academic and operating agencies. The term of each appointee would be two years. No one discipline would dominate, but rather a multidisciplinary point of view would be maintained. Flexibility and easy access to university and state agency authorities would be accommodated. A high premium would be given to the issues of public and mental health, i.e., chronic mental illness, the two-class system of care, and explication of the relationship between need, manpower, and technology.

The First Experience

In his interim report after the first year, Dr. Prevost wrote:

> The basic approach for changing behaviors between the two sectors would be the application of the sociological axium that interaction promotes the development of common norms. Mutual tasks and problem-solving would therefore characterize the endeavor. (4)

Ten strategies were initially identified and developed by Dr. Prevost. They provide a sense of how he saw the system and the strategies necessary to address the issues. These strategies included:

1. Beginning trust
2. The development of mutual priorities
3. Maintenance of existing relationships
4. Intrasystem liaison
5. Don't do it yourself
6. Transfer of relevent knowledge into service practice
7. Merging operational service responsibilities
8. The focus on psychiatry
9. Bridging constructs
10. Sustaining momentum

December, 1984, marked the completion of the first Galt Scholar's incumbancy. The products of this first efforts were considerable.

1. A formal contract exists between each of the Departments of Psychiatry and the Department of Mental Health and Mental Retardation's three largest state mental hospitals.

2. Special clinical evaluation units have been established at two of the state hospitals.

3. An insulated state hospital residency program has been changed. Through affiliation, university faculty members are available formally to teach in the hospital. Residents have the opportunities of attending seminars and lectures at the medical school. All three state hospitals now have active exchanges and affiliations between university residency programs and hospital staff.

4. Formal research activities have been established. (5,6)

5. Recruitment of well-credentialed professionals, including a director of one of the state hospitals, has been established.

6. Several mental health manpower studies within the department have been completed.

7. A general sense of partnership and identity between the three Departments of Psychiatry and the Department of Mental Health and Mental Retardation has been established.

Implications for the Future

The new Galt Scholar, King Davis, Ph.D., a tenured professor in the School of Social Work at Virginia Commonwealth University, assumed his position in January, 1985. There was some concern on the part of the chairmen that this disciplinary shift may alter the close collaboration that has grown over the first years between the departments of psychiatry and the State Department of Mental Health and Mental Retardation.

There is legitimacy to some of this concern. Broadening the base of participation to include another discipline will, of course, alter the rhythm of the relationship that Dr. Prevost, a psychiatrist, developed in his tenure as the Galt Scholar. But as Dr. Prevost bridged the State Department of Mental Health and Mental Retardation and the three departments of psychiatry, so the next bridge will be between the different disciplines and the State Department of Mental Health and Mental Retardation. There is no question that the major mental health disciplines have, in an important sense, drawn together their different orientations to become dominated by a private, office-based, psychotherapeutic practice.   In social work, for example, fewer and fewer graduates are going into public agency practice.   And even fewer are practicing in programs dealing with the social dimension of chronic illness, or with the people who have chronic mental illness. (7)

This homogenization across disciplines has been costly. It occurs, ironically, at a time when psycho-social programs for chronic mentally ill persons have demonstrated their effectiveness and utility.

The next phase of the Galt Scholar's task will be to address the increased distancing of collective mental health disciplines from public programs, and from chronic mental illness. It will explore ways to encourage each discipline to examine its own technical base, as well as the relationship of this base to other disciplines. The common point of reference will be chronic mental illness.   The bridging, therefore, will facilitate an understanding of the multiple needs of persons who are chronically mentally ill. It will also facilitate an understanding of the needs of the practice system - especially those practice pieces which address the professional concern for those who are seriously mentally ill.

In his final report, Dr. Prevost wrote: "The Galt Scholar position because of its location in both the service and academic systems is appropriately owned by neither. Nor does the position have any assigned staff or for that matter, authority. Responsibilities remain the broad goals of the agreement between the Department of Mental Health and Mental Retardation and Virginia's three universities with medical schools as described in the first report. While all of this at first may seem to describe a poorly constructed position, further thought and experience support the wisdom of the initial role conceptualization. The Galt Scholar's loyalty is to the goals of both systems and the development of collaboration between them. How to be this intermediary and agent of change is left to the ingenuity of each two-year incumbent thus assuring fresh views and approaches to complicated systems issues.   The levers of the Galt Scholar are contingent and relative rather then organizationally constant thus requiring change but assuring relevancy. The leverage is that of access to the leaders of the two systems with the expectation that the Galt Scholar will persuade and negotiate behaviors consistent with the goals of the agreement. Assuring this opportunity to influence could not occur if the position were viewed as in one camp rather than the other or possessing authority over resources. (8)

Conclusion

The Galt Scholar program has been a success. It has directly addressed a difficult set of problems and provided a framework against which to examine the relationship between the three publicly supported universities and the State Department of Mental Health and Mental Retardation. This has included three different state hospitals as well as a department-operated treatment center for children. The legislative resolution of 1982 has been honored by all parties.

A major accomplishment has been the recognition that the public mental health system cannot be separated from the academic system. There is a mutuality of need that goes beyond resources. It is a need that goes beyond turf and a guild mentality. It is the recognition of a common enterprise, an enterprise that refuses to accept a two-class system of care. And further, the successful elimination of a two-class system requires the active partnership of the university and the public mental health authority.

Over two hundred years have passed since 1773, when James Galt was appointed "Keeper" of Eastern State Hospital in Williamsburg, Virginia. The professionalism that this family provided lasted until 1880. The course of time through our own day has seen incredible change for chronically mentally ill people. It has been a history of failure and success on a grand scale. As we turn more and more toward the twenty-first century, the Galt Scholar and its vision will enable us to learn from the past; and in pursuing knowledge, research and service, the focus on serious mental illness will be the commonwealth of both the university and the service agencies. It is from this relationship that the success or failure of our disciplines will be judged.

REFERENCES

1. Dain N: "Disordered Minds: The First Century of Eastern State Hospital in Williamsburg, Virginia, 1766-1866". Charlottesville, University Phase of Virginia, 1971

2. 1982 Regular Session Engrossed House Joint Resolution 112, Feb 10, Virginia 1982

3. Galt Visiting Scholar in Public Mental Health Agreement" effective January 1, 1983

4. Prevost JA: "The Galt Visiting Scholar Chair in Public Health, Interim Report: A Review of the Beginning Year, Feb 1, 1984 (unpublished paper)

5. Vieweg V, Rowe W, David J, et al: Hyposthenuria as a marker for self-induced water intoxication and schizophrenic disorders. Am J Psychiatry, 141: 1258-1260, 1984

6. Vieweg V, Rowe WT, David JJ, et al: The "Mini-Mental State" examination in the syndrome of self induced water intoxication and schizophrenic disorders (SIWIS): a pilot study. Int J Psychiatry Med 14(4), 1984

7. Robin A: Community Mental Health in the Social Work Curriculum, New York, Council on Social Work Education, 1979

8. Prevost JA: The Galt Visiting Scholar Chair in Public Mental Health: Report for the Year 1984, Nov 20, 1984 (unpublished paper)

WHAT CAN GO WRONG WILL – AND DID:
THE EMORY–GEORGIA EXPERIENCE

Jerry M. Wiener, M.D.

Long, long ago in a land far away, a University Department of Psychiatry (UDP) and a State Department of Mental Hygiene (SDMH) entered into a relationship with each other. UDP entered, at least in large part, on the expectation of a handsome dowry, but sincerely intending to be a faithful partner. SDMH thought of it more as an arms-length affair, rather expensive perhaps, but not requiring fidelity or a promise of longevity. SDMH's parent (the State) was not ungenerous to UDP in providing an elegant home named the Georgia Mental Health Institute (GMHI) and a generous annual allowance, but from the beginning SDMH was ambivalent about the union and withheld its affection. UDP's parent (the University Medical Center) seemed pleased primarily to have transferred financial responsibility for one of its children and was more concerned that the marriage not be dissolved, even if preserved in name only. As is often the case in such marriages, it was the offspring, e.g., Child Psychiatry (CP), who in the long run ended up suffering the most. Other offspring also were affected, including the general residency training program, interdisciplinary collaboration, the quality of clinical care, and to a lesser degree, the research program. However, Child Psychiatry suffered the most immediate and perhaps long-term damage. The issues in this relationship will be examined primarily from the writer's perspective during the time he served as director of child and adolescent psychiatry in the Emory department of psychiatry and concurrently as director of the division of youth (children and adolescents) at GMHI.

The reader should know beforehand that in the writer's judgment, this is a story on the State side of good intentions in high places miscarried by simplistic assumptions; and on the University side, of policies more concerned with academic appearances than academic priorities. The story begins with high hopes and great expectations; it ends with the gutting of the substance of a state-university training/research/service relationship, while preserving its outer shell. The drama of the relationship contains elements of political intrigue, personality conflicts, philosophical differences, interdisciplinary rivalries, and even the influence of religion. It will be organized, as befits the introductory analogy, in sections of Courtship, Honeymoon, Estrangement, Separation, Aftermath and Post-Mortem.

Courtship

In 1964, the State of Georgia and Emory University (through its department of psychiatry) agreed on a collaboration at the Georgia Mental Health Institute (GMHI). This facility provided a large and modern central administration/teaching/research building surrounded by spacious and separate treatment units, including one each for adolescents and children. Modeled initially on the concept of the New York State Psychiatric Institute/Columbia University relationship, GMHI was to be the principal training and research flagship for both the department of psychiatry and the state.

The Emory UDP was to provide both administrative and professional direction. This academic affiliation and leadership was intended to attract and retain a high quality of clinical and research staff, offer a model of clinical excellence and innovative services in a public institution, and provide for the training and retention of young professionals in the state and in the public system. The chairman of the department of psychiatry at Emory also was to be the superintendent of GMHI, thereby creating a more perfect union.

However, even before GMHI opened, there was discord. The SDMH was opposed to relinquishing so much control over such an important facility and so large a budget, so it was agreed that the superintendent would be appointed by the state to be responsible for administration, service delivery, and non-medical training. The chairman of the department of psychiatry at Emory would have the right of approval on the appointment of the superintendent, control of research faculty appointments, direction of psychiatric training, and would appoint unit chiefs jointly with the superintendent. The unit chiefs would be responsible to the superintendent for services and to the chairman for training, and hold full-time faculty appointments at Emory. Residents were appointed by Emory; stipends were provided by the state. Under these terms, the marriage was agreed to (consummated might be too strong a word).

As already indicated, from the beginning there were snakes in this Garden of Eden. The director of SDMH was perceived as an unsympathetic and meddlesome in-law. The directors of training in the other mental health disciplines (psychology, social work, chaplaincy, etc.) resented Emory's favored position and control of faculty, and battled for autonomy and equality.   However, the facility itself was elegant, the overall budget was generous, and Lester Maddox was governor – so there were other things for people to worry about.

Honeymoon

In 1971, I arrived as the new director of child and adolescent psychiatry at Emory and concurrently as director of the youth division at GMHI. The two positions were considered essentially as one. I was recruited by the chairman, and approval of my appointment by the superintendent at GMHI was described as more or less pro forma. The entire Emory Child and Adolescent Program – offices, clinical facilities, faculty, staff and budget – was housed at GMHI, with the exception of a small but promising service at Grady Hospital, the city-county public hospital affiliated with the medical school as its major teaching site for the clinical departments.   It was understood that at GMHI, the director of the youth division would be co-equal to the medical director for adult services, who was also full-time Emory faculty (i.e., the money came from the GMHI state budget, but the paycheck was issued at Emory).   In response to my concerns, assurances were provided of the right of the UDP chairman to approve the appointment of the superintendent at GMHI. In this way, Emory always would be able to assure that a superintendent would be appointed who was sympathetic with the objectives of the affiliation. This reassurance was accepted at face value, and the position accepted.

In the first one and one-half years, significant progress was made in building the Child and Adolescent Programs. An academic faculty and staff were recruited for the GMHI and Emory-Grady Programs. Both the career-training program and child psychiatry training for general residents were reorganized. Soon, there were more qualified applicants for career training than could be accepted.

The only full-range clinical service for both children and adolescents in the state was established at GMHI and included inpatient, day hospital, special education, and outpatient therapeutic services. Outreach consultation services to community agencies and child-care facilities were begun, and trainees rotated to Grady Hospital for experience in a general hospital setting with an inner-city population and consultation/liaison with pediatrics. The relationships between the superintendent at GMHI, the chairman, and the director of the youth division facilitated this growth through collaboration on the basis of clear guidelines, open communication, and shared priorities.

Estrangement

In 1972, then Governor Jimmy Carter embarked on a badly needed reorganization of an anachronistic state mental health system. A new director of mental hygiene for the state was selected, and a well-meaning, but young and inexperienced lawyer with close political ties to the governor was appointed chairman of the board of human resources.

Battle lines were quickly drawn between the administrative and legislative branches, between the new liberal populists and the entrenched conservative establishment, between urban and rural constituencies, between what some called the "New South" and the "Old South." Storm clouds quickly gathered over GMHI.

The superintendent, a nationally respected psychiatrist/administrator, soon found himself at odds with the new director of mental hygiene over both philosophy and plans for GMHI, and resigned under pressure. A new superintendent was appointed in early 1973 without prior consultation with the Emory chairman. This superintendent had held a staff position in the New York State Department of Mental Hygiene; he was not a psychiatrist, not a clinician, and had not had prior experience in a program which combined training, research, and clinical service delivery. He did, however, have a "philosophy," consistent with the times, which fit well with the populist identity of the administration and the objectives of the new SDMH director. This new director of mental hygiene was a psychiatrist who had received most of his own training in a state hospital, and so far as could be determined, had little experience with university training programs, research, or clinical practice after his residency.

The director and the superintendent had served together in the New York State Department of Mental Hygiene, and brought with them their personal version of the then prevalent "community mental health" movement, which included the following principles (implicitly or explicitly):

1. Services should be "decentralized," and decision-making should be as "local" as possible.

2. Except for legal requirements, the professional disciplines should be relatively interchangeable. Usually social workers, psychologists, nurses, ministers, and others were preferable to psychiatrists because they cost less and did not believe in vertical hierarchies. This point was important because without it, given the state's limited number of psychiatrists, the first goal of decentralization was unattainable. The requirement that unit chiefs at GMHI be psychiatrists was unilaterally terminated.

3. It was unilaterally decided that GMHI should be only one of the several regional hospitals in the state system, serving a geographic catchment area of several counties. Like other regional hospitals in the "new" state system, its role as a hospital would be one of last resort, and it would be accorded no special consideration as a training and research center.

4. It was critical to assume that the greater availability of community-based services would significantly decrease the need for hospitalization, so that hospital staff could be redistributed to community-based services. Apparently it was never considered that better local services would identify even more cases of serious psychiatric illness.

5. The "community" was where services were to be delivered, so that was where training should be conducted. Training in general at GMHI was viewed as secondary to decentralized service delivery, and even more, training in psychiatry per se was considered important only so far as it supported the new decentralized delivery system.

6. Any questions, differences, or simple presentations of facts were considered self-serving "elitism" - the dying gasp as it were, of an outmoded medical (versus social) model.

7. Consistent with all the above, the premium was on training "mental health generalists" who would be able to take care of most of the problems of most people. Specialist training and practice was deemed an unnecessary and elitist luxury. (The superintendent was reported as stating that people would not have mental illness if they were more religious.)

8. In declaring the end of any "closed" wards or units at GMHI, the superintendent expressed his philosophy in the following quotes (from a memo) ". . . if a physician declares that a patient cannot be treated in a facility lacking a closed ward he is simply displaying ignorance of what is being done in progressive facilities . . ." and ". . . it would be impossible for anyone to escape from GMHI because no one is to be incarcerated." These statements were made when GMHI was the designated regional state hospital serving a population of several hundred thousand people, many of whom were committed to GMHI in accordance with state law and/or were brought by police officials because of behavior harmful to self and/or others.

Conflict, both overt and covert, quickly developed among the new superintendent, the director of the youth division, and the chairman of the department. Prior agreements regarding administrative policy, medical staff organization, admission procedures, staffing levels, budget, and the definition of role and responsibilities were all arbitrarily swept away by one administrative fiat after another.

Most were made without prior planning or consultation, and without prior notification of the unit chiefs and division directors involved, specifically in the youth division. Many were made within hours or days of explicit personal commitments or reassurances to the contrary by the superintendent.

The entire basis on which GMHI had become a major training resource for the Emory psychiatry residency program was radically altered within a period of a few months. This was particularly true in child psychiatry.

The chairman seemed powerless to influence these events. Appeals to the director of the state system were futile; the chairman of the board of human resources (who had ultimate legal authority) had little option but to back the governor's appointee. With the exception of but a few members, officials of the local and state mental health associations seemed completely enamored of what seemed to them actions achieving the desirable goals of decentralization, deprofessionalization (especially of psychiatry), destigmatization, community-based services, and "human services" programs (replacing the objectionable "medical model").

The legislature was locked in battle with the governor over many issues, and the fate of GMHI and its university relationship seemed important only as a political football. The local and state psychiatric societies protested vigorously, but too often in a way that was perceived (occasionally accurately) as only self-serving. The small child psychiatry community, almost all of whom practiced in Atlanta, was vigorous and vehement in its expression of concern, but was too small a constituency to have any significant impact in a highly politicized environment.

For the first several months, almost the entire professional and support staff in the children's and the adolescent units at GMHI remained remarkably loyal and cohesive. However, at the central administrative level there were intense interdisciplinary conflicts and maneuvering for power: covert and anti-university attitudes became overt and vociferous; the relationship between clinical services and training needs almost ceased to exist; the atmosphere was pervaded by conflict, tension, mistrust, anger, accusations, distortion, and political cabals.

In April, 1973, the director of the adolescent unit resigned. In May, the youth division director recruited and selected a replacement who was to have a full-time Emory appointment approved by the chairman. This person was then refused an appointment by the superintendent.

In early November, 1972, the superintendent informed the Emory chairman by memo that the position of "deputy superintendent for youth" (as it was then called) was abolished effective immediately, leaving the position responsible only for child psychiatry training. All service and administrative responsibilities were shifted to the "deputy superintendent-medical" (an individual also holding an Emory full-time faculty appointment who was loyal to the chairman but acquiesced in, if he did not encourage this action).   At no time did the superintendent discuss with or even inform the director of the youth division of this decision, not even by copy of his memo.

The chairman and dean of the medical school also acquiesced in this action, citing their helplessness to act otherwise because of the financial dependence of the department on GMHI.   In January, 1974 (two months later), the chairman responded by memo to the superintendent's action, reporting to him that the department's executive committee had met on November 14, 1973 and expressed its opposition to the action.   Unfortunately by January, 1974, the action was a fait accompli, and the protest was an empty gesture.

Separation

Following the superintendent's action, alternative plans had to be made.   The former deputy superintendent for youth remained director of training in child and adolescent psychiatry at GMHI until June, 1974 in order to honor obligations to the child psychiatry trainees and faculty who had been recruited to GMHI.   By July, 1974 a modest outpatient service and faculty offices were established at Emory to serve as a home base for the division of child and adolescent psychiatry.   (It should be noted that the chairman was most supportive in helping to provide the space and a small operating budget.)   The Grady Hospital Service (always operating on a shoestring budget), the Henrietta Eggelston Hospital for Children on the Emory campus, and a local investor–owned psychiatric hospital were developed as new training sites.

The director of the children's unit and the adolescent unit at GMHI resigned (both were board certified child psychiatrists), as did the chief social worker, the chief nurses and several other staff members.   What had been the only program in the state of Georgia offering a full range of quality services and training in all mental health disciplines quickly disintegrated into a "decentralized" and stereotypic state hospital program.

Instead of remaining in the public sector, child psychiatrists entered private practice and the for-profit hospital system.   Instead of continuing in the direction of increasing excellence and national prominence, the training programs in both child and general psychiatry became limited almost entirely to either local recruitment or less competitive applicants. The Emory department of psychiatry as a whole underwent a period of faculty turn-over and demoralization. The services for children and adolescents (as well as for adults) at GMHI underwent a period of destabilization, lack of leadership, deprofessionalization, and difficulty recruiting and retaining psychiatrists.

Aftermath

By mid-1974, there was so much turmoil and disaffection in the state system as a whole that the board of human resources recommended and the governor acted to dismiss the director of mental hygiene, who was the governor's own appointee and architect of the new state system. In 1976, the superintendent of GMHI resigned. In December, 1975, the director of child and adolescent psychiatry at Emory (and formerly the director of the youth division at GMHI) resigned to accept an academic position in another state. In 1974, the governor's term in office expired; by state law he could not succeed himself. In November, 1976, he was elected President of the United States. In June, 1982, the chairman of the department of psychiatry at Emory retired.

Post-Mortem

A state-university relationship which serves the interests of both is clearly possible - other chapters in this volume describe successful joint ventures of mutual benefit. What can and did go wrong in one such venture has been described in this chapter. What were the reasons?

First, there must be a clear definition of the responsibilities and priorities each side brings to the partnership. The academic health center's first priority is to provide education and training to medical students and residents, a responsibility usually delegated and implemented through an organization of basic and clinical science departments. Its second priority is to conduct research both for scientific advancement and as an enrichment to education. Patient care is necessary and indivisible from the education and research missions. One cannot conceive of medical student education, residency training, and clinical research (or of retaining faculty or fiscal solvency) without quality patient care. However, patient care, and even more so "service delivery systems," are not unique academic health center responsibilities, except to the extent that they support educational and research missions.

The state, on the other hand, ultimately and traditionally has a primary responsibility for the delivery of services within the public health and mental health systems. It collects taxes for this purpose and is accountable to its citizens. However, the state also may see the support of medical and postgraduate training as important to fulfill and/or enrich its service delivery responsibility, and of both general and specific benefit to its citizens.

Given that the academic health center must have clinical facilities and patients to provide for its education and training missions and that the state has a significant patient care responsibility, a partnership may well serve the needs of both. Each must retain sufficient control to fulfill requirements of responsibility and accountability: the university over education and training, the state over service delivery and patient care. Each must genuinely value the benefits provided by the other, and must respect the priorities, politics, and value systems of the other (e.g., state appointment and civil service policies versus the university faculty/academic value system).

Agreement to collaborate in overlapping training, research and patient care activities must reflect and not assume or ignore the above areas of understanding and mutual respect.

Under the best of circumstances, any state-university relationship is bound to encounter periods of tension, political pressures, changes in personnel on both sides, fluctuations in the economy, budgetary concerns, and perceptions by both sides that the other is gaining or taking advantage. Any agreement must provide for mechanisms and procedures to deal with these sources of tensions; and must provide structures and support for sufficient continuity and longevity to buffer the program from short-term pressures and the political appointment process.

With these principles in mind, the most salient reasons why this state-university relationship ended in conflict and friction may be summarized:

1. From the beginning, there was ambivalance on the state's part about the relationship, and there was no effective state-university mechanism for addressing differences or changes.

2. There was insufficient investment and commitment to the relationship on the part of the university. The health center did not view the relationship primarily as an opportunity for collaboration which would supplement and enrich its programs in psychiatric education and research. The department of psychiatry ultimately found itself without any clinical or training base in the medical center or university hospital, and therefore without any leverage when pressures began to be applied by the state.

3. There was never a firm joint commitment by both the state administrative and legislative branches to the GMHI contract, so it quickly could become a political football rather than politically protected.

4. A new state administration made a needed decision to completely reorganize its mental health delivery system emphasizing decentralization, regionalization, deprofessionalization, and a non-medical "human services" concept of "mental health" services. A new director of mental hygiene (a psychiatrist who had no prior training or experience in or with an academic health center) and a superintendent of GMHI (a non-clinician) were appointed to implement the new system, with little or no regard for either the special identity and mission originally intended for GMHI or for the impact on considerations important to training, and with little awareness and/or concern for the connection between quality services and quality training.

5. The department, while early on viewing these appointments and their consequences with alarm

and concern, more or less acquiesced rather than overtly articulating its valid reasons for concern and opposition and working actively to influence the system. It was thought that behind-the-scenes political maneuvering combined with the appearance of cooperation would allow for damage control at an acceptable level. The judgment of the department that there would be little support from the medical center administration in such a struggle was probably correct.

6. Latent or barely covert interdisciplinary conflicts over issues of status, control, and autonomy were exascerbated and exploited, rather than moderated and contained.

7. Finally, there were personality, attitudinal, and motivational conflicts which went beyond either philosophy or politics, although they were rationalized in philosophical and political terms. While these always are present to some extent, the climate and events described above prevented their resolution. Perhaps in the final analysis, it was this most-of-all human dimension which was the most destablizing if not destructive element.

STATE-UNIVERSITY COLLABORATIONS:
WHY DO SOME FAIL?

James T. Barter, M.D.

Donald G. Langsley, M.D.

A number of papers have been written recently describing the virtues of state-university collaboration in
training, research, and service (1,2,3,4).   Advantages of
such collaborations from a university standpoint have
included: expansion of training programs into public sector
settings; a source of revenue to support training programs;
new part-time faculty at small additional cost; opportunity
to teach continuity of care; and access to stable cohorts of
patients for research (5,6).   Advantages from the state's
standpoint have included: better patient care; improved
quality of state training programs; increased prestige for
programs leading to enhanced staff morale and increased
retention; and easier recruitment of qualified faculty and
staff (7,8).

The success of programs such as those in Maryland
(1,9), and Oregon (10,11), and the obvious advantages of
successful collaborations for both parties have tended to
obscure the difficulties inherent in trying to bring two
bureaucracies together into a joint venture. This chapter
will focus on the authors' knowledge of successful collaborative programs as well as those which eventually fail.
The roots of such failure and the general principles underlying these dissolutions may serve to point out ways of
avoiding similar disappointment in existing programs.

The authors, separately and together, have been instrumental in developing programs which involved public
sector/university collaboration. Some of these programs
were successful for a period of time and then came un-
raveled. Four programs will be described briefly; some of
the reasons for their eventual failure or success will be
suggested, and the general principles elucidated.

Describing the complex interplay between all the
political, social, behavioral, historical, and other factors
which played a part in the success and failure of these
programs is beyond the scope of this chapter. We have
selected our data arbitrarily; these are our ideas about
what happened. We realize that other observers might
offer alternative explanations; however, we believe the
principles derived would be similar.

UC-Davis/Sacramento County

In 1968, the County of Sacramento and the UC-Davis
Department of Psychiatry entered into a collaborative
agreement. Under the terms of this agreement, the

Department of Psychiatry would assume administrative leadership of the County Mental Health Program (the Chair of the Department of Psychiatry served as the County Mental Health Director). The Department also would be responsible for recruitment of psychiatrists and other mental health personnel (there were 13 vacant psychiatrist positions which the county-run program had been unable to recruit). More importantly, there was a significant commitment to provide direct and comprehensive mental health services for large segments of the county for which prior services were less than optimal. Sacramento County obtained a university-run comprehensive mental health program from this collaborative venture. The University obtained stable funding from the county Short-Doyle budget, which permitted rapid growth of a fledging department. Other advantages were similar to those described in the introduction.

From 1968 to 1973, there was a rapid growth of the program. The university operated the only 24-hour psychiatric emergency service and thus controlled the triage of acutely ill persons to mental health services. Services were organized by catchment area and expanded. The university initiated operation of three community mental health centers, effectively decentralizing most outpatient and aftercare services. Continuity of care was assured by making each center responsible for outpatient, inpatient, and aftercare services. Staff vacancies were filled, and over 20 new psychiatrists were recruited into the community.

A psychiatric residency program was started which eventually grew to include 40 residents. All residents had essentially similar training within the community mental health programs; there was no separate university training track. A few residents spent a year at one of the state hospitals as part of a separate contract with the state for support of training.

Among the accomplishments in this time period was a marked reduction in the numbers of patients being sent to state hospitals, from 90 per month to less than five. Some of the funds saved by not sending patients to state hospitals were made available for community programs. Chronic patients were served from the beginning of the program. There was a massive increase in outpatient visits, from less than 7,000 per year to over 75,000 per year. Most of the graduates expressed a decided preference for public sector psychiatry, and over 90% of graduated psychiatrists went to work in public sector settings (12,13,14).

Initially, both the university and county expressed satisfaction with the contractual arrangements. A master agreement covered details of mutual responsibility and accountability between the two. A separate contract was negotiated each year which was linked to the annual mental health plan required by the state. This latter spelled out levels of expenditure, new program initiatives, staffing levels, and other day to day details.

There was a separate agreement between the county and the university covering general medical care for indigent patients. The county hospital was jointly operated by the county and the university. By agreement, mental health was treated separately from this contract for other hospital services.

In 1972, the university negotiated the purchase of the county hospital for use as the university teaching hospital. The county contracted with the university to continue providing care for medically indigent persons. Contract negotiations were arduous and at times, acrimonious. This reflected the concern of both the county and university that the other was attempting to secure unfair advantage in the medical services contract, and also was stimulated by the retirement of the county hospital administrator who had been instrumental in promoting the university-county collaboration, as well as the county's appointment of a newly formed unified health agency director who was committed to showing the county supervisors how much money he could save.

The university's purchase of the hospital led to a shift in direction of the county mental health program. The county came to be fearful that if the university continued to direct mental health, there would be a loss of accountability, and valuable service dollars would be subverted for educational and research purposes. Both the master mental health agreement and the specific year to year contracts were rewritten. In contrast to prior year contracts, the new contracts were more tightly written with more specific constraints, and could be construed as being imbued with a higher degree of distrust of each party's motives.

From 1973 on, the county assumed direction of the mental health program and contracted with the university for delivery of services at approximately the same level as before.   The senior author (JTB) replaced the second author (DGL) as mental health director but maintained his university base and commitment. Because both believed in the value of university and county collaboration, there were no major changes in the character of the program. There was, however, a heightened level of scrutiny of the mental health program by the county governing body and more need to justify the continued reliance on the university as the major contractor for mental health services. This change was reflected in a decline in the percentage of the county mental health budget which was allocated to the university programs, even though total dollars remained generally constant. New program monies generally went to contractors other than the university. Throughout this period of time there were disputes between the university and the county about the medical services program.   In addition, accusations began to surface that the university mental health program was inordinately expensive because of the inclusion of training costs as part of patient treatment costs.

There was also a marked increase in consumer group pressure for "a piece of the pie." Specialized groups, dealing with drugs, alcoholism, orthomolecular approaches, and similar single interests, with the support of the county mental health advisory board, were able to convince the county governing board to fund their programs preferentially.

In 1976, there was a change in chairs of the department of psychiatry. The new chairman's priorities were not as firmly wedded to maintenance of a public/university cooperative effort. In addition, the county/university contract dispute over medical services became less cordial. There was a demand for a reassessment of the mental health agreement as part of the overall university/county agreement.

In 1976, the county mental health director (JTB) resigned, weary of the political pressures and the ability of local groups with special interests of their own to gain direct access to the county governing board.

Over the next two years, there were increased demands for accountability of the mental health program. Accusations about high cost of services became more prevalent. The county governing board seemed less and less satisfied with the agreement, and there was considerable sentiment for seeking alternative methods for delivering mental health services. A study of the university mental health program was commissioned in an atmosphere of increased acrimony. University officials who heretofore had treated mental health as separate from the general medical services agreement sought to link the two in the belief that the county would fear losing the university-provided mental health services, and thus, would grant concessions in the medical services' contract.

The commissioned study was highly critical. Errors and omissions in the study went unchallenged by the university. The end result was the county's decision to decrease significantly university participation in the delivery of mental health services. By 1979, the university was essentially out of the provision of mental health services for the county. Most of the decentralized mental health centers were closed, and centralization of services was dictated by the problems of adequately staffing the centers, the low status of working for these county-operated programs, and assumptions about the need to adapt to limited resources.

The university training program underwent a series of reductions to less than half its former size, as it became impossible to fund or provide suitable training sites for a large program. There were drastic cuts in faculty and staff, and reorganization of the program into a "typical" university training program. A model public sector/university mental health collaborative program had ceased to exist.

University of Cincinnati/State of Ohio Cooperative Program Proposal

In 1976, one of us (DGL) became Chairman of the Department of Psychiatry at the University of Cincinnati. This prestigious university program had a long tradition of training psychoanalytically oriented psychiatrists. Many of its graduates traditionally gravitated toward academic careers. The cutback in national training funds and general academic support made the possibility of a state-university collaboration attractive. In addition, broadening the training opportunities to include public psychiatry was consistent with the personal bias and commitment of the new chairman. A proposal for a state/university collaborative program was developed.

Several factors were considered to be favorable for such a proposal. The close proximity of two state institutions, one a state hospital and the other a state psychiatric institute with significant research potential, enhanced the attractiveness of cooperation in training, research, and service. The state authorities were receptive to this collaboration and saw many advantages accruing to the two institutions. The university administration was similarly receptive.

The major stumbling block was the department of psychiatry faculty who feared dilution of the existing program. This faculty placed a lesser value on public psychiatry training and were reluctant to commit their time and energy to making the program work. There was mistrust of the intentions of the affiliation agreement, an unwillingness to participate in development of mutual priorities and merge operational service responsibilities. In the end, the faculty's suspicion and distrust doomed the proposal to failure.

State/University Cooperative Training Program

In 1977, the director of health for the state of California became concerned about the loss of psychiatrists from the state hospital system to community programs and expressed interest in making these institutions more attractive places in which to work. He also was interested in improving the quality of the existing training programs in state hospitals. University affiliation was viewed as an appropriate strategy to accomplish these goals.

In 1978, one of us (JTB) became involved in trying to promote cooperative training ventures between state hospitals in California and selected campuses of the University of California. This project had its origin in a study of state hospitals which came to the conclusion that free-standing state hospital training programs could be enhanced by formal affiliation agreements with university training programs (15). It was asserted that such affiliations would result in better staff morale, improved recruitment and retention of staff, and stimulation of relevant research activity.

Although this project started off with a great deal of enthusiasm and pledges of commitment from the deans of medical schools, the state had problems focusing priorities. Partially, this problem was a result of the confusion

attendant on the state breaking up the massive consolidated health department, resulting in newly formed
departments of mental health and developmental
disabilities.   The former director of health had a
commitment to the project; the new director of mental
health gave it a lower priority.

One concrete result of this project was the
development of a contract involving the University of
California at Davis (UCD), Napa State Hospital (NSH) and
the State Department of Mental Health (DMH).   This
contract was initially envisioned as one in which the
university would assume total responsibility for the
operation of the psychiatry residency training program at
NSH. This proposal immediately ran into resistance from
NSH officials who valued the independence of their training program and felt it was a major source of trained
personnel for the hospital. They were suspicious of the
motives of the university. DMH wanted the affiliation but
was unwilling to mandate the change. The UCD was willing to consider the affiliation and operate a combined and
integrated program but was concerned about the 55-mile
distance between sites. The eventual compromise was that
the DMH agreed to pick up the training costs for a select
number of UCD residents each year in exchange for having
all residents in the UCD program rotate through NSH.
Because of continued suspiciousness and resistance at NSH,
the two programs were functionally separate, with
residents from UCD doing their training on wards separate
from the NSH residents and having a separate seminar
schedule as well as separate supervisors.

The program was difficult to implement. UCD residents resisted going to the state hospital, and they were
aware of the tensions between the programs. UCD faculty
were similarly reluctant to make the long drive to NSH to
carry out training and supervision of a few residents. In
spite of the initial difficulties, many of the residents
eventually saw the rotation as a positive training
experience. In the end, the lack of progress toward any
integration, coupled with DMH budgetary problems led to a
gradual defunding of the program and its demise after
three years.

University of Colorado–State of Colorado Collaboration

We also are familiar with the university/state collaborative program at Colorado. It began in the mid-sixties when the state hospital at Pueblo (110 miles from the residency program in Denver) had difficulty in recruiting and retaining psychiatrists. The chairman of the department of psychiatry at Colorado viewed the opportunity to collaborate as enhancing the department's visibility with the state legislature which provided significant training funds to the university program. The state hospital welcomed the collaboration, since residents would spend one or two years at the hospital, and since a major part of the educational program involved full-time university faculty who would travel at least once weekly from Denver to Pueblo. The residents enjoyed the experience, because of the higher salary they were paid, and because they were given a gratifying role and experience at the hospital. In that setting, they were given authority to establish and operate units or programs of their own, and the supervision given was seen as nurturing that role. The residents in a five-year program would spend a year at Pueblo between the first and second year of training and after the fourth year. Those on the four-year program, had only one year at Pueblo.

Residents at Pueblo felt linked to the Denver program by virtue of the weekly contact with senior faculty who made the trips. A number of Pueblo psychiatrists who were not part of the residency program came to Denver regularly for brief clinical experiences, grand rounds, or other educational opportunities.

The Denver–Pueblo program was born and fostered in an atmosphere of mutual trust and support. It was enthusiastically supported by both the chairman and the senior faculty at Denver and by the superintendent and senior staff at Pueblo. Communication was effectively enhanced by regular contacts and close liaison carried on by the training director. There was little or no sense of a two-class system, nor did the university avoid its awareness of service responsibility in return for the economic advantages offered by the state.

Discussion

These examples illustrate many of the pitfalls inherent in trying to establish and maintain state (public)/ university collaborative efforts. It is possible to derive from these experiences some principles which seem guaranteed to promote failure of such affiliations.

1.   Foster Suspicion and Mistrust

When one or both parties to an agreement distrusts the motives of the other, then one can assume it will be impossible to initiate a workable contract. Furthermore, projects which may have been operating smoothly can be disrupted by suitable injection of suspicion and mistrust. This sense of suspicion and mistrust can and, usually, has to be mutual to operate effectively.   Sacramento County's distrust of the university, and the university's certainty that the county was trying to take unfair advantage played a significant role in the eventual loss of university provision of county mental health services. Mistrust of the department chairman's motives in Cincinnati led to a failure to develop the affiliation agreement. A similar climate of distrust prevented the achievement of an integrated university training program between UCD and NSH.

2.   Maintain Separate Priorities

Universities and public programs have quite different missions.   These differences result in formation of separate priorities. Insistence on maintenance of these separate priorities can assure that a workable collaboration will not be realized. In order to scuttle collaborative agreements, universities need only to eschew any interest in public service or agree only to the most limited public service role possible. In a similar fashion, public programs need to see only the service needs of the populations being served and steadfastly refuse to support education or research as politically unwise or as an illegal subsidy of educational programs.

3.   Ignore Existing Relationships

A sure fire recipe for failure is for both public programs and universities to ignore existing relationships. This is particularly important at times of leadership change. Often relationships are established between two parties at the onset of a working agreement which fosters collaboration; over time, there are leadership changes, and less attention is paid to nurturing the ongoing relationship. The new leaders, not having been involved in the initiation of the program, do not feel the same sense of commitment to the program as did the initiators. Certainly a factor in the ultimate dissolution of the contract between Sacramento County and UCD was the departure of the chairman of the department of psychiatry and a year later, the resignation of the county mental health director. The new chair and new county mental health director may have assumed that the existence of a renewable contract was sufficient to keep the program viable. An outside observer would have noted a deterioration in personal relationships between the county mental health personnel and the university staff during the last three years of the contract.

4.   Ignore Formalized Liaison Relationships

Formalized liaison relationships between cooperating agencies tend to provide a structured channel for communication and conflict resolution. Failure to set up such formalized liaisons, or refusal of one or another party to agree to such formalized relationships results in increased distancing, a sense of isolation, and insufficient time to work through issues with eventual increased friction. In the Napa State Hospital/UC-Davis agreement, the lack of formalized liaison between the university and the state hospital resulted in crises meetings during which mutual grievances were aired but rarely resolved.

5.   Go Your Own Way

The essence of cooperation is compromise. Insistence upon going one's own way weakens or destroys collaborative efforts. In the examples cited, there were factions who insisted upon maintaining separateness. Some of the University of Cincinnati faculty could see little or no advantage to a state collaborative program and pursued their own independent agendas. During the last three years of the UC-Davis/Sacramento County contract, political forces in both the county and the university could see more supposed advantages to maintaining separateness than they could to continued cooperation. NSH's insistence on maintaining its program as a separate unaffiliated entity and the university's acceptance of academic apartheid sowed the seeds of eventual failure.

6.   Keep Operational Service Responsibilities Separate

The idealized state/university collaboration in mental health merges operational service responsibilities. One can assure failure by making sure that there is at least a two-tiered system of services, one of which is considered to be an elite, academic, psychiatric service program serving selected patients, and the other for public patients, with complex intake procedures, long waiting lists, low staff morale, inadequate facilities, and poor administration.

7.   Promote an Antimedical Model of Mental Health

University training programs in psychiatry are often accused by "mental health advocates" of excessive devotion to a "medical model." Public programs, on the other hand, are frequently seen as espousing a "social disability" model of mental illness. This polarization leads to failure to agree on program goals and ultimately to poor collaboration. University psychiatry training programs exist within medical schools and train physicians in psychiatric medicine; additionally many programs teach from a comprehensive biopsychosocial model of psychiatric illness. To insist upon an antimedical model of public mental health services as a condition of collaboration leads to failure.

The university programs in Sacramento County were seen as being "excessively medical," a factor which was also alleged to promote excessive cost of treatment services. Advocates on the mental health advisory board used this accusation as a rationale for decreasing the size of the university contract responsibility in favor of social rehabilitation model programs with little or no medical input.

8. Establish Ambiguous Administrative Roles

Not knowing who is in charge of what and making everyone in charge of everything are administrative principles which lead to chaos. Similarly, establishing ambiguous administrative roles between two cooperating bureaucracies leads to confusion, lack of accountability, and loss of direction. Contracts which fail to spell out clear administrative roles for each of the collaborating agencies assure failure.

While none of the examples in this paper suffered from this particular principle, it is so basic a fault that it needs to be mentioned.

Discussion and Summary

We have presented case examples drawn from our experience of why some state/university collaborative mental health programs can fail. We do not mean to imply malevolence of any person or agency involved. It is important to keep in mind that some of these examples had degrees of success. Certainly the Sacramento County - UC-Davis mental health program was imaginative, innovative, and demonstrated a nationally recognized model of cooperation for a period of time. The UCD - NSH residency rotation was a good training experience for those who participated. The kind of agreement which it represented is not uncommon. Many state hospitals serve as settings for rotation of university psychiatry residents without their parent department or chairman having an administrative role in the state hospital program. The Cincinnati program, which never got beyond the proposal stage, was an attempt to broaden the base of support for the department while assisting the state programs.

What is sobering is the discrepancy between the amount of effort that is required to initiate and develop a collaborative program and that which is required to bring about its demise. Even carefully constructed contractual agreements can be dissolved rapidly when both parties are tired of the arrangement, or feel that the other party has gotten much the better part of the deal.

Even though our principles are stated in the negative, what to do if you want to make a program fail, it is easy to turn them around and derive positive principles for success. Many of these principles, positively stated, have been cited in papers attempting to elucidate what is

necessary for successful collaborative effort. We chose
this form of presentation to fix the reader's attention on
how common such mistakes can be. It is a dramatic rather
than a sophistic device.

REFERENCES

1. Harbin HT, Weintraub W, Nyman GW, et al: Psychiatric manpower and public mental health: Maryland's experience. Hosp Community Psychiatry 33:277-281, 1982

2. Faulkner LR, Rankin RM, Eaton JS Jr, et al: The state hospital as a setting for residency education. J Psychiatr Education 7:153-166, 1983

3. Faulkner LR, Eaton JS Jr, Bloom JD, et al: The CMHC as a setting for residency education. Community Ment Health J, 18:3-10, 1982

4. Greenblatt M: University-hospital collaboration in psychiatric education. Ment Hosp 16:167-169, 1965

5. Faulkner LR, Eaton JS Jr, Rankin RM: Administrative relationships between state hospitals and academic psychiatry departments. Am J Psychiatry 140:898-901, 1983

6. Faulkner LR, Eaton JS Jr: Administrative relationships between community mental health centers and academic psychiatry departments. Am J Psychiatry 136: 1040-1044, 1979

7. Garver KD, Norman ML, Greenblatt M: Life at the state summit: views and experiences of 18 psychiatric leaders. Hosp Community Psychiatry 35:233-238, 1984

8. Ash P, Knesper DJ: Influence from psychiatric education on subsequent career choice: with special reference to work in state mental hospitals and the shift to private practice. J Psychiatr Education 5:285-294, 1981

9. Weintraub W, Harbin HT, Book J, et al: The Maryland plan for recruiting psychiatrists into public service. Am J Psychiatry 141:91-94, 1984

10. Cutler DL, Bloom JD, Shore JH: Training psychiatrists to work with community support systems for chronically mentally ill persons. Am J Psychiatry 138:98-101, 1981

11. Cutler DL, Terwillinger W, Faulkner L, et al: Disseminating the principles of a community support program. Hosp Community Psychiatry 35:51-55, 1984

12. Barter JT: Sacramento county's experience with community care. Hosp Community Psychiatry 26:587-588, 1975

13. Spensley JS, Werme PH, Barter JT, et al: LPS and the mental health center. California Med 114:49-51, 1971

14. Langsley DG, Barter JT, Yarvis RM: Deinstitutionalization - the Sacramento story. Compr Psychiatry 19:479-490, 1978

15. Kurtz WJ, Merwin EP, Nielsen S: State hospital recruitment and retention program: prepared for the Director, California State Department of Health, 1978 (unpublished report)

PITFALLS OF JOINT VENTURES BETWEEN STATE AND ACADEMIC INSTITUTIONS: THE NEW YORK EXPERIENCE

Sheldon Gaylin, M.D.

Erica Loutsch, M.D.

In general, any cooperative venture between two large and complex organizations is likely to have some unexpected, often disappointing results.   To the extent that the organization's goals and the parameters of mutual responsibility in a cooperative venture are not clear, the potential for failure increases dramatically.   There are a variety of general situations, with pitfalls for the unwary, which occur so frequently in joint ventures that they deserve a review in a volume such as this.

In this chapter, we will describe the administrative, political, social, and attitudinal issues that create difficulties in cooperative ventures between state and academic institutions, using the experience in New York State as a paradigm.

The New York State Department of Mental Health and its relationship to the academic community has been selected as our prototype because the authors have had numerous, frequently frustrating, but often rewarding experiences working with (and within) the state system.   In addition, the Department of Mental Health of New York State makes an ideal case study of the pitfalls in cooperative ventures between state government and academia, because New York has always been among those progressive states that strive to provide the best services for the mentally ill.

Albert Deutsch acknowledged New York State's leadership role in his book, The Mentally Ill in America: "The evolution of state care. . . in the United States followed a long and winding trail before reaching its most significant expression with the passage of the New York State Care Act of 1890." (1)

The authors polled a small group of distinguished academic psychiatrists who have broad experience with state governments.*   All agreed that service, research, and

---

*   The authors would like to thank the following for their comments and suggestions: Kenneth Altshuler, M.D., Professor and Chairman, Department of Psychiatry, Southwestern Medical School; Haroutun M. Babigian, M.D., Professor and Chairman, Psychiatrist-in-Chief, Department of Psychiatry, The University of Rochester Medical Center; Fritz A. Henn, Ph.D., M.D., Professor and Chairman, Department of Psychiatry and Behavioral Science, State University of New York at Stony Brook; Marvin I. Herz, M.D., Professor and Chairman, Department

education are legitimate goals both of state facilities and academic institutions.   Where, then, are the areas of conflict?

The conflict occurs primarily in the ordering of these goals - service, research, and education. It is not simply a question of semantics. Careful attention must be paid to the competing priorities. While no one element is inherently more important to society than the other, government facilities and academic departments of psychiatry, by legislation or common understanding, assign a higher priority to one over the other.

Although the priorities of both state institutions and academic departments of psychiatry include patient care, research, and teaching, their ordering of these priorities definitely differs. The state institutions generally see their primary function as patient care, with research directed toward improvement of that care and prevention of illness and disability. Educational functions are necessary to maintain their staffs' clinical skills. Academic departments of psychiatry, on the other hand, have the mandate to teach medical and other advanced students, and to expand basic knowledge in the field of behavioral science. Critical to both mandates is the provision of good patient care.

There are invariably problematic consequences resulting from these differing priorities. In state institutions, the unrelenting obligation to provide patient care may interfere with even rudimentary research and teaching. Academic facilities typically do, and indeed should, limit patient care to a level that will maximally support teaching and research programs. Outside pressures also dictate, to a large extent, the behavior of the institutions. Any academic department of psychiatry which allows its research and training operation to decline because of pressure to provide quality care will soon hear from its peers and those responsible for assuring academic excellence. At the same time, any state facility which permits its clinical services to fall below acceptable standards must sooner or later face an outraged public.

The state system is, of course, responsible to the public. The interpretation of what society desires in its public programs is usually left to elected officials who, at the very least, must face the collective wish of society at election time. The problem, however, is that government officials do not necessarily have a direct line to the heart of society's wishes.

A clear statement of how to define society's wishes for public programs has been made by one chairman of a department of psychiatry, who observed the continuing commitment of tax dollars publicly and openly is the only true determinant of what society wants to support. (2) By this definition, both academic departments of psychiatry and state departments of mental health currently are faring very poorly indeed.

In an ideal world, all the goals - education, research and patient care - would receive appropriate funding in both kinds of institutions. But in the real world, resources are always limited. The question then becomes which goals will be compromised. Academic institutions, in general, respond to severe limitations of resources by reducing the amount of service provided on a selective basis, and by maintaining maximum resources in those areas which are best suited to teaching or research purposes. Government-sponsored programs, in the face of restrictions, attempt to maintain all services on an egalitarian basis, regardless of teaching and research needs.

When the existence of different priorities of the two kinds of institutions is not clearly acknowledged, trouble invariably develops. The typical consequence of the failure squarely to confront legitimate differences in institutional goals is the use of moral arguments and/or vague language to obscure difficult administrative issues.

One such example occurred during the early 1960's, at a time of great pressure to shift responsibility for the care of the mentally ill to local communities, without the corresponding shift of financial resources. It was during this time that the term, "major mental illness," first became fashionable in the speeches and writings of members of the New York Department of Mental Health. There were constant complaints that local mental health services, including academic departments of psychiatry, would not deal with the "major mental illnesses." The implication was that community agencies were not doing their share in dealing with the most important problems. "Major mental illness" was never defined. The department of mental health tended to use the phrase to define disorders that were so serious that they required hospitalization in state facilities. This circuitous argument probably postponed for many years legitimate study of the role a state hospital system might play in caring for the chronically ill, as compared to the role that community agencies might assume for the same population.

An example of the use of moral or pejorative arguments to avoid resolving the difficult problems of serving two distinctly different mandates is the complaint that academic institutions are not interested in serving the most needy population, although there is a moral responsibility to do so. Academic institutions are often pictured as selfishly or self-centeredly serving the "worried well" and the "deserving rich," while state mental health facilities must serve all individuals with serious mental illnesses.

Since it is the policy of the State of New York that all of its residents who are disabled will receive care, the state is forced to, and indeed does, take care of many patients who are rejected by other institutions. Despite the great reduction in patient population due to deinstitutionalization (75% since 1955), the restriction in admissions of geriatric patients, and the emphasis on short-term hospitalization, the main characteristics of the state hospital population remain today the same as they were in Dorothea Dix' time. Most state hospital patients are the severely and chronically mentally ill - with a great majority from the lower socio-economic groups. State hospitals continue to be the setting of last resort. Despite the growth of community resources, community mental health centers, psychiatric units in general hospitals and private psychiatric hospitals, there is a group of patients for whom these programs are unable to provide adequately: the actively aggressive, the court-referred criminal, the assaultive, the severely mentally retarded, and the one-third of the schizophrenics who never recover in spite of the efforts at treatment. Even newly established state hospitals which began without chronic patients are beginning to experience a buildup in long-stay patients, especially those with histories of violent or dangerous behaviors, mental retardation and psychiatric illness, or those under criminal court proceedings. (3)

Due to changes in policies and definitions of mental illness, the state hospitals even have had to accommodate persons with alcoholism and drug addiction and those previously contained in the criminal system. The increase in alcoholics, drug addicts and criminally adjudicated patients, who are mostly young and male, and the decrease in elderly patients needing only custodial care has changed the sex ratio to more male than female. All of these factors force the state hospitals to provide a wide variety of programs for the most dangerous and chronic populations. (4)

Goldman et al describe the state hospitals currently as providing short-term, intermediate and long-term care, voluntary and involuntary custody (in 1979, only half of the patients were voluntary admissions) to predominantly disadvantaged persons, with the most severe chronic and acute mental disorders - those patients that are unacceptable or inappropriate for other settings. The state system thus, is the asylum of last resort - "where the buck stops." (5)

Often, mandated services are grafted on the existing programs with inadequate facilities and staff, and this has distressing effects on all services, old and new. The lag between legislative mandates and the funds to support the resulting programs tends to be more of a problem in states where new programs are mandated to meet political pressure, and those states, such as New York, in which the courts are active in adjudicating long-standing unresolved problems. It is the policy of the State of New York that all of its residents who are disabled will receive service according to individualized needs. (6,7)

How does this policy affect the academic institutions? While public policy assigns responsibility to state facilities for care of last resort, this responsibility does not relieve the academic community of its defined obligation to expand knowledge in behavioral sciences and communicate new findings. Persons who are chronically ill, criminally insane, or multiply disabled, etc., are of great public concern, and these conditions are fertile areas for research and training programs, providing obvious ground for cooperative ventures between state institutions and academia while each maintains its priorities. As long as government does not provide funds for these patients to be treated under the purview of the academic institutions, then the academic institution should play a leadership role in encouraging government to provide the funds for research and education related to problems associated with these difficult issues, while not assuming the patient care responsibility of the state hospital system.

Even the effort by a willing and prestigious academic department to assume a leadership role in teaching and research in community psychiatry, while providing opportunities to improve its relationships to the community, can lead to failure when conflicting goals and priorities are not clarified.   The development of the Community Mental Health Center in the Washington Heights–Inwood section of Manhattan in the mid-1960's is a relevant example. This was essentially a federal–state funded project, part of the massive Community Mental Health Centers Development Program when state versus federal rights issues were dominant. New York State at that time was the acknowledged proponent of state authority in mental health, and there were major battles between New York City and the federal government on one side, and state government on the other, in the development of the community mental health centers programs in New York City. It was the responsibility of the director of the Columbia University Mental Health Center project, a member of the academic department of Columbia University, to negotiate the development of the Mental Health Center in the Washington Heights–Inwood section of Manhattan. The service area originally was to extend from 155th Street north to the end of Manhattan Island.

The department of psychiatry's academic goals were to develop a model service program under the Community Mental Health Services Act and to utilize this program for teaching and research, while at the same time to expand the department's activities into areas which had been long-term interests, such as social psychiatry, epidemiology, and public health. A community mental health center was seen as a logical extension of the pioneering community and administrative psychiatry program which had been established for many years as a joint venture of the school of public health and the department of psychiatry. The integration of a large government-funded program allowed for major academic growth. The department's representative permitted primary academic concerns for teaching and research in community psychiatry to be subverted by the lure of the availability of major new facilities with attendant opportunities to increase staff. This led to rationalization and acceptance of decisions that ignored basic concepts of community organization and clinical development.

The department accepted the city's decision to enlarge the program to include the community from 125th Street north, which expanded the population served to over 400,000 and combined the predominantly black and Hispanic community below 155th Street with a lower middle-class Jewish and Irish-Catholic district above 155th Street. Federal representatives insisted that if the facility were to serve separate communities, it must have two separate entrances - one designated for the Inwood section, the predominantly white area, and the other designated for the 125th Street section, the predominantly black and Hispanic population. The obvious implication of separate black and white entrances fell on deaf ears. Meanwhile, the constant struggle between state and federal and local governments made it impossible to pay attention to the desires of the community, which ultimately rejected the entire project. In retrospect, it appears that outcome was appropriate, although at the time, it was a painful experience for all involved. Here was a classic, if unfortunate, example of what happens when neither institution is paying attention to its primary goals and responsibilities.

Sometimes, the true objectives and/or priorities of an institution are not made explicit for a number of reasons. Staff members may know civil service regulations, but choose to ignore them. Academicians and state hospital personnel often insist that they are forced to make vague or secret arrangements in order to avoid fruitless confrontations with unnecessarily rigid state bureaucracies. The concept that government service requires a higher standard of ethics, but not trust, leads to extensive checking and counter-checking, often costing more than the anticipated savings. (8) Academic and non-academic clinicians alike often spend a high percentage of their time justifying the cost of clinical care, which reduces the energy and time needed to provide quality care, research, and education. Paradoxically, the approach often stimulates in those receiving government benefits the sense that, since there is neither trust nor honor expected, none will be given, further fostering the rationalization that government deserves to be cheated when it can be cheated - always an inappropriate conclusion.

An example of the sort of difficulties that can occur when this attitude prevails is seen in the following excerpt from the report of the auditor-general of a large Eastern state. The report concerned the activities of a physician, a "full-time, salaried employee . . . (who) also serves on the staff of a major medical center and hospital and is compensated modestly for his time as a part-time salaried instructor." This individual was criticized for "conducting educational classes at the . . . (state institution) . . . during regular scheduled working hours, primarily for psychiatric residents and psychology interns of the medical center." The criticism continued that he, ". . .with authorization of the superintendent, directed employees under his supervision to type, on state time, three different drafts of a clinical case review. A final draft of this project fulfilled part of the requirement for the clinical director's training to become a certified psychoanalyst." In addition, "The clinical director, from time to time, assigned state employees clerical duties for two professional organizations with which he is affiliated. The employees, using state time and property, typed, photocopied, and mailed correspondence to members of organizations, and typed minutes of meetings when the clinical director was secretary of the professional organization. Correspondence to the organizational members was mailed nationally and internationally. Records at . . . (the state hospital) . . . indicated over a period of two months alone, $80.00 in state funds were expended to mail correspondence of the clinical director to places such as Switzerland, Argentina, and Canada, where members resided." (9)

Clearly, these activities might well be encouraged for some members of an academic department of psychiatry. However, the rules of most civil service positions would declare these activities questionable, if not illegal, unless specifically spelled out in the individual's job description. In this particular situation, it seems likely that the individuals involved knew the civil service rules, but chose to risk a potential disaster in order to avoid the confrontations and compromises that might have occurred when negotiating the original contract. Either that, or they chose to employ the rationalization that the system deserved to be cheated.

New York State law no longer refers to the "indigent and pauperized insane," yet there is a tacit acceptance of a different level of care. (10) When an academic institution contractually accepts this concept of a lower standard of teaching, research, or patient care within a state facility, trouble arises. Less talented teachers or clinicians are assigned; seminars and lectures are geared to the lowest level of sophistication. Medical students and residents, if they are assigned at all, are often sent with the attitude of observing the way a system should not operate, or simply to provide basic services at minimum levels. There is an implication that the affiliation is a necessary evil to secure additional funding for training and research activities.

Senior academic psychiatrists are well aware of the problems of working with the state or federal bureaucracy. Many of the chairmen of medical school departments of psychiatry have had such experiences. A large and diversified literature documents many of the problems encountered. At the same time, we are aware of only one article alluding to the abuse of state facilities by academic institutions. (11)

We believe there is a need to enlist the academic community's support for public programs for the mentally ill as a natural extension of the community's prime mandates. Two of the pitfalls, pervasive in the relationship between state facilities and academic institutions, are the acceptance of a lower standard of care, teaching, and research for those who work and are treated within state facilities, along with the assumption that any of these activities can be done more cheaply at the state facility than at the academic institutions.

There are a number of pitfalls to be avoided in any joint venture between state and academic institutions, and most problem areas are immediately apparent upon inspection of proposed or actual contractual agreements. A contract which accepts a lower quality of care, research, or training in a state facility is always a mistake. A contract which allows higher academic rank for the staff at a state facility than otherwise would be warranted by their academic credentials is always a mistake. A contract that specifies payment for service to be defined at a later date is always a mistake.

What is important in order to avoid such pitfalls? The acceptance of the mandates of training, research, and service as legitimate functions of both the state facility and the academic department of psychiatry is but the first step in the development of cooperative and productive relationships between these two institutions.

Cooperative ventures must be undertaken with open agreements among equals with respect for the responsibilities and rights of each partner, the limitations of the other.

In addition, academicians must stop thinking of the state bureaucracy as a natural enemy. Bureaucracy is defined as ". . . government by bureaus, usually officialism." (12) The central function of a bureaucracy - the need to assure continuous operation in the face of major political or social changes - is essential to both organizations.   It is the resistance to change, the bureaucracy's stickiness despite all outside efforts to move it, that gives bureaucratic behavior its more pejorative meaning of obstructionism, pettifogging, and rigidity. Large academic and government institutions share many characteristics of bureaucratic organizations. When either group attempts to initiate significant changes in core activities, the bureacracy tends to interfere with these changes, slowing them down and sometimes blocking them entirely. The academician, primarily, feels blocked by the governmental bureaucracy because of the perceived need to make changes in the primary concern of the state hospital system - service to patients.   It makes little difference that the utlimate goal in such changes in the system would be improvement in the service system as well as the academic teaching and research programs. If the roles were reversed, and the first attack were made upon the education of medical students, skewing it toward providing additional service to the state hospitals, one would find an equally fierce response from the bureau-cracies inherent in the medical education system.

The most successful long-term cooperative ventures between state facilities and academic institutions have been the simple purchase of educational services. Recent information suggests that 75% or more of all academic facilities have such arrangements with state facilities, and both sides seem to be satisfied. (13)   These relationships tend to be well defined in advance, with limited goals and no hidden agendas.

The problem situations we have described - doing good by cheating, subverting programs for important but unagreed upon goals, purchasing academic appointments, acquiescing to unacceptably lower standards in state facilities, are symptoms of two underlying problems: a lack of attention to the effects of competing priorities and the acceptance of a double standard of care for the mentally ill.

With rare exceptions, the academic community has done little to utilize its educational and research strengths to expose and correct this inequity, and the state facility community has not had the strength to mobilize the political and administrative support to protect itself and its patients.

As one department chairman said to a commissioner of mental health some years ago, "It is a difficult process, but we should be heavily involved together, not because if we are successful, it will be of benefit to both of us, but because it is the right thing to do." (14)

REFERENCES

1. Deutsch A: The Mentally Ill in America. New York, Columbia University Press 1949, p 229

2. Michels R: personal communication

3. Sheets JL, Prevost JL, Reihman J: Young adult chronic patients: three hypothesized subgroups. Hosp Community Psychiatry 33: 197-203, 1982

4. Peele R, Lipkin J: Public mental hospitals, in Psychiatric Administration: A Comprehensive Text. Edited by Talbott JA, Kaplan SR. for the Clinic Executive, New York Grune & Stratton, 1983

5. Goldman HH, Taube CA, Regier DA, et al: The multiple functions of the state mental hospital, Am J Psychiatry 140: 296-300, 1983

6. Preamble and legislative findings for 1977 reorganization of department of mental hygiene, L-1977: C.978 1, effective April 2, 1978, McKinney's Consolidated Laws of New York, Annotated, Book 34A, Mental Hygiene Law, p3

7. Ibid, paragraph 7.01, p 22

8. Talbott JA: The problems and potential roles of state mental hospitals, in State Mental Hospitals: Problems and Potentials, Edited by Talbott JA. New York Human Sciences Press, 1980, pp. 25-26

9. Anonymous mimeographed report

10. New York Laws of 1980, Chapter 126

11. Zwerling I: The public hospital system as a nexus between government and the university, in State Mental Hospitals: Problems and Potentials, Edited by Talbott JA. New York Human Sciences Press, 1980

12. Compact Edition of the Oxford English Dictionary Oxford, Oxford University Press, 1971

13. Faulkner L, Eaton J Jr, Rankin R: Administrative relationships between state hospitals and academic psychiatry departments, Am J Psychiatry 140: 898–901, 1983

14. Miller A, quoting Milton Rosenbaum, M.D., personal communication

THE ANATOMY OF A DEVELOPING RESIDENCY PROGRAM 1964–1984

Walter W. Winslow, M.D.

Introduction: Background and the Development of the Physical Plant

In 1964, the University of New Mexico School of Medicine matriculated its first class of 24 students. Soon after, most major departments began developing residency training programs. The school of medicine has expanded, but is still a small school with 73 undergraduate students each year and over 150 house officers in training in various specialties of medicine.

In the early years of the department of psychiatry, the highest priority of its faculty was development of quality clinical programs to provide an adequate base to teach and train medical students and psychiatric residents. Initally (1964), the department had an 18-bed ward in a university-county hospital, a small outpatient clinic in temporary quarters, and a Veterans Administration Hospital that was preparing to increase its psychiatry service from eight to 48 beds. In 1969, a Mental Health Center (MHC), operated by the university, opened its 44 adult inpatient beds, four satellite outpatient clinics, a partial hospital program, and a 24-hour crisis service. The 18 beds in the university-county hospital were closed, and except for a consultation-liaison service, all psychiatric services for the entire medical center were to be provided by the MHC.

The MHC was built on the University of New Mexico Center campus with $800,000 from county bond money matched by a federal construction grant. In 1966, the Veterans Administration Hospital opened its renovated 48-bed adult inpatient psychiatric service to complement the partial hospital, mental hygiene clinic, and consultation-liaison programs. In 1976, construction began on a 53-bed Children's Psychiatric Hospital (CPH), also on the medical campus. This institution also is operated by the University of New Mexico.

In 1977, the MHC was asked by the city, county, and state to take over a city/county alcoholism and drug abuse treatment program. This change added 20 alcoholism treatment beds, and outpatient programs for treatment of alcoholism and drug abuse.

In 1983, the MHC, with county bond money constructed a 30-bed addition to the inpatient unit: 15 beds for adolescents and 15 beds for geriatric patients.

In 1978, a child and adolescent division was organized within the department of psychiatry, and a child psychiatry fellowship program was developed soon thereafter.

In a period of less than 20 years, the department has put together an array of programs and institutions adequate for the education and training of medical students, psychiatric residents, and child fellows, as well as providing other elements necessary to an academic department of psychiatry.

Development of a Faculty

In 1963, the first chairman (Dr. Robert Senescu), who was one of the first six faculty members employed by the University of New Mexico Medical School, joined the dean in the process of building a medical school. In 1966, I joined the faculty and worked closely with Dr. Senescu in the planning and building of the department's faculty, facilities and programs. In 1970, I was appointed director of the MHC, and in 1974, I was appointed chairman. The department faculty has grown over the years, its members staffing the various institutions in the medical center (university hospital-consultation/liaison, MHC, VA Hospital, Children's Psychiatric Hospital and the Child Guidance Center) and now consists of 45 tenure track faculty, 45 full-time faculty on a clinical track and approximately 30 clinical (voluntary) faculty (Table I). The medical school has had three deans since 1963; the present dean has held this position since 1971.

Funding of Stipends for Residents in Training

In 1966, we accepted our first resident, a staff physician at the state hospital who wished to have training in psychiatry. His stipend was paid by the state hospital all three years of his training, the first and last such support from the state hospital. In 1967, the department obtained NIMH Basic Residency and General Practice Training Grants.

In the early years of the program, these NIMH grants provided the major portion of the stipend support with additional support from the VA Hospital and the university-county hospital. For example, in 1969-1970, of the nine positions filled, four were paid from this Basic Residency-NIMH grant, three from the GP Residency-

NIMH grant, one from the VAH, and one from the state hospital.

By comparison, in 1975-1976, when most of the NIMH support was discontinued, of the 20 positions, two were Basic Residency-NIMH, seven were VAH, 9.5 were from the mental health center, and 1.5 from the university-county hospital. As the federal grant support for stipends was phased out, the stipend support was picked up by the MHC and the CPH. For example, in 1983-1984, out of the 29 positions filled, the VAH funded six, the MHC 19, the CPH 1.5, the UNM Hospital 1.5, and one was funded by the Minority Fellowship Program of NIMH (Tables II and III). The Children's Psychiatric Hospital also funded three child fellow positions. We are presently evaluating the need for further program growth, and it seems unlikely we will increase beyond 30 positions for the general residency program. However, there is planned growth in child psychiatry, to three fellows in each year. Fifth year fellowships in geropsychiatry, forensic psychiatry, and substance abuse are under consideration.

Where Do the Graduates Practice?

Since 1966, 82 residents have participated in the program; 68 have graduated. Some left the program to go into other specialties, and a few were dropped for poor performance. Thirty-one (45.5%) of those graduated have remained in New Mexico; 22 are in private practice; one is employed by the state hospital; and eight are on the faculty of the department of psychiatry at the University of New Mexico.

Influencing Factors: Internal and External

As all training directors and chairmen are aware, the internal allocation of funds for stipends in a medical center (including the VA) is a very complex process based as much on relationships, credibility, and clout with the dean, the director of graduate education, hospital administrators, and others, as on rational argument. The ability to locate stipend support for a growing program from other sources was of particular importance in the 1970's when NIMH support was gradually being phased out. Not only did we have to find new sources of stipend support for growth, but at the same time, we had to find funds to replace lost NIMH support. Our strategy was to seek new stipends from the mental health center, the Children's Psychiatric Hospital and support from various outlying community mental health centers. This proved to be a very uncertain option since CMHC's were undergoing their own funding difficulties in the 1970's with their federal funds also rapidly diminishing. In our case, during the 1970's, with a good management team in place, our university-operated mental health center was sufficiently stable and fiscally sound to be able to begin and gradually increase its support of residency training. As chairman and director of the mental health center, I had easy access to the center's board of trustees. This gave me many opportunities to discuss with them the value of supporting residents' stipends. Getting stipend support from the Children's Psychiatric Hospital which is primarily state funded was a little more difficult, since it was necessary to obtain "line item" funds specifically for training residents and child fellows from the legislative and executive branches of state government. This approach required meetings with key legislators and cabinet level leaders in state government. Again, this was not only a rational process but also a political one, with considerable time needed to educate key people in state government and in the legislature regarding our needs. The process required numerous trips to the state capitol, attendance at many committee meetings, interacting with key individuals, not just during the legislative session but throughout the year. The support of the dean who is most adroit at working with the legislative and executive branches of state government was of inestimable value in this process. Similar efforts were necessary with city, county and state governments for increasing support of our growing clinical programs which, in turn, strengthened them financially and allowed them to develop into good quality training sites.

Discussion

I.   What were the key factors that made it possible to increase local support for stipends when national support was being withdrawn?

A. Long-term relationship with the dean and other key university administrators.

B. Long term relationship with the MHC board of trustees and the board of regents of the University of New Mexico.

C. The university's willingness to permit the development of a medical school and medical center to operate service programs for the city, county, and state. This set the tone for good working relationships with the city, county, and state governments.

D. Stability in the department and the dean's office. The dean has been in office since 1971; I have been director of the MHC since 1970, and chairman since 1974.

E. Ability to develop long lasting relationships with key state legislators, city councilmen and county commissioners. (One county commissioner who was a good friend later became a strong supporter of mental health in the state legislature.)

F. Willingness of the chairman and other faculty members to serve on community committees, councils, task forces, and boards. These activities provided the department with visibility which was of great help during the legislative process.

G. Long and short-range planning. Having strategic plans for a changing environment coupled with a long-range plan is essential.

H. Political instincts (inherited or developed). The ability to work with, not against, the political process in its many forms is essential as is the need continually to refine these skills.

II.   What are the risks and problems in this process?

A.   May become too politicized. Political "foes" as well as political "friends" have long memories. Your gains (successes) may be viewed as others' losses (failures).

B.   Time involved. Many hours on a year-long basis are required to develop and keep alive the relationships necessary to develop visibility and credibility, the basic ingredients necessary for success.

C.   Failure to do homework. Appearing before a committee to testify is sometimes only a formality, but it must be done well. However, the outcome may be dependent upon the informal contacts prior to the formal presentation. (Much is still accomplished in "smoke-filled" rooms, with less smoke these days.)

D.   "Burn out." Political networking can only be partly delegated to your assistants. It requires your personal attention. Sometimes a team of two or three individuals can be developed, but this requires careful coordination. The risk of "burn out" is high.

Summary

The task of developing and maintaining mental health institutions in an academic medical center for education, research, and service is only a little more difficult than developing and maintaining stipend support for residents from various constituencies including federal, state and local public authorities and health care institutions. It requires abilities to work not only with the internal politics of the academic medical center, but also with political forces at all levels of government. This process may be enhanced in a milieu where the chairman, the dean, and other key administrators have relatively long tenures, where their views and goals are often congruent and where each has a well developed political network. Community visibility and credibility also are essential ingredients.

Having a long-range plan, regularly updated, and having a team capable of developing strategies for various contingencies are essential to the success of any organization and no less important in the development of stable funding for a residency program.

And lastly, not to demean the collective efforts of all those who contributed to the success of the program during difficult times, I am unable to assess objectively the impact of elements such as accidental good timing, extraneous or fortuitous events, or just plain luck as significant factors contributing to our success.

ACADEMIC PSYCHIATRY AND "THE PUBLIC SYSTEM": A POINT OF VIEW

Milton H. Miller, M.D.

While it is possible to offer plausible explanations for events by proposing a causality that is not flesh and blood and very personal, such explanations are usually wrong. The wish, the plan, the determination of a particular individual or group of individuals has a lot to do with what happens in real life. "I decided," "we decided" is regularly the key ingredient in the chain of events that leads to something special. At least, that's how it has seemed to me during these last three decades of my career as psychiatrist, teacher, and administrator. For example, I have found that many successful education and human service programs, and the administrative arrangements supporting such undertakings don't translate well in second or third locations. The reason is that it is never "just a program" that achieves success, it's "a program into which life and direction have been breathed by ....." and no less, "a program right for this time and this place." This is not to suggest that Ayn Rand, the 1940's author of Fountainhead and Atlas Shrugged (1,2), was completely correct in annointing rugged individualism as the only source of creative achievement. The general environment greatly influences human undertakings. But, individual values are very important, and so is the matter of the intensity with which values are put into practice. Important also is the matter of who it is who believes strongly in something. In particular, it helps a great deal if the boss really believes in the job.

What follows is a brief discussion of the complexities involved when an academic psychiatric program and a major public care system found their destinies inexorably intertwined, i.e., if the academic program failed, the public system failed! And vice versa! Simultaneously, a model is described in which one individual or group of individuals assumes responsibility for "excellence" both in academic psychiatry and in major public mental health programs. Specifically, the chapter will detail the problems and promise associated with a mental health system where the professor and chairman in several UCLA-affiliated psychiatric departments serves also as deputy director, Los Angeles County Department of Mental Health with responsibility for catchments of 1.5-2.2 million people. In particular, I will draw from my own six years of experience in the combined posts of professor and chairman of psychiatry at Harbor-UCLA Medical Center and director, Coastal Region, Los Angeles County Department of Mental Health.

The decision to unite academic and public care programs rests upon a set of institutional and personal priorities, and this chapter begins with a statement of assumptions and values that underlie the administrative arrangements in our system.   But after the values have been declared and a mode of implementation has been planned, the realities of the actual bringing to life of the idea inevitably provide new perspective.   Does the theory work in real life?   What is the cost?   As a partial answer, this chapter will provide a description of the kind of effort that has been necessary in Los Angeles to create an effective melding of public and academic programs during a time when there was a terrible defunding of public systems because of California's Proposition 13 (decreased local tax revenues) and the substantial early 1980's national downturn in the economy.   Discussion will also include detailing the benefits, including "fringe benefits," of melding public-academic psychiatric concerns.   They included, in Los Angeles: a) the very survival of both the academic and public care systems during a critically stressful interval, and b) unique opportunities for research, special training, and other clinical experiences that came because there was <u>trust</u> between the two sectors.

Basic Assumptions and a Personal Historical Perspective

Functionally   discrete   "academic,"   "public,"   and "private" sectors of American psychiatry exist in many cities and states.   Despite the overlapping activity of individual clinicians and shared membership in local socieities and the American Psychiatric Association, it is the absence of assistance rendered and the failure to plan together which characterizes many of our professional communities.

This substantial separation is a very serious problem, one which for decades has weakened all parts of our profession, diminishing our effectiveness in serving our patients, their families and society.

One of the most serious effects of the divisions within psychiatry is that "no one," or worse, "someone else" is responsible for the deficiencies that exist in all sectors of mental health care. Individual clinicians think of themselves as "doing a good job" even though "the system is bad."

My own personal perspective on the matter of "public is public," "private is private," and "academic is academic" changed from casual acceptance to genuine concern in 1974. I had been a professor for 20 years and a chairman of academic departments for 12 of those years. Even earlier, my teachers in Topeka, Kansas, Karl and William Menninger (3,4), had espoused a psychiatry that would always turn toward the sickest, most neglected parts of our society. Still, it required a sojourn to a nation in South Asia to make me personally critical of the attitude that one could think highly of self and the division of the profession in which one worked even if the overall mental health delivery system wasn't so good. I was working as a World Health Organization consultant to a country with many millions of people. Most of those millions had little or no general medical care. The country was poor. But beyond poverty, there was an almost total separation of private doctors, academic doctors, and the government's health officials and doctors. Even within the separate groups, there were major divisions. In the larger cities where there were several medical schools with psychiatry departments, each department had its own residents all of whom had narrow and inadequate training. Combining efforts between the programs, however, seemed impossible. They were little fiefdoms. In general, the universities were elitist in that poor country. The tiny public mental health system was hostile to university and private caregivers, each of whom in turn, was hostile or indifferent to the other. The result was catastrophic for millions and millions of people, mediocre education for all the young, and an opportunity for an outsider like myself to be very critical. And everybody blamed "the other."

When I came home and thought about certain similarities in health care deficiencies in that poor nation and in my own, I felt ashamed. We have fewer excuses (5).

Do Academics Share Responsibility for the "System?"

Work with the seriously mentally ill public patient has regularly subjected the caregivers to the same prejudice and neglect that the patients themselves have received (6). So, a certain amount of vision and idealism as well as a long-term perspective are necessary in such work. Its importance is unquestioned. But the problem exists for the caregivers for public patients and poses dilemmas for psychiatric educators who have a dual responsibility:

1. The teachers need to make the young feel a personal commitment to make our mental health system work for <u>everybody</u>.

2. Equally, we have a responsibility to protect young physicians from squandering their invaluable training years in what has often been a hopeless quagmire of underfunded and defunded public services for the chronically and severely mentally ill. "Too much service" (especially at the expense of learning) is the other name for public psychiatry.

In theory, it should be possible to match clinical situations with trainee needs. In real life, however, that blending is often quite difficult. Many prestigious psychiatric training programs have little or no affiliations with public mental health programs. Often, psychiatric education programs in larger communities divide into those which are primarily concerned with public mental health systems and those which have no public patient responsibility whatsoever. In Los Angeles, half the psychiatric residents have vastly too much public patient concentration, whereas the other trainees have, in my judgment, too little of the kind of experience that teaches: <u>I</u> share responsibility for the care of <u>all</u> psychiatry's patients.

In the Los Angeles academic community during the period between 1976 and 1983, those portions of the academic system closely associated with public patients, primarily the Los Angeles County University of Southern California Medical Center and Los Angeles County Harbor-UCLA Medical Center have experienced extraordinary stress. At Harbor, resident recruitment was made very difficult, and morale became a serious problem: the drain on everyone has been constant and intense. The primary reason was that a flood of desperately sick public patients continued to arrive at County Harbor-UCLA Hospital though the resources for their care were rapidly dwindling. Seven thousand patients annually arrived in the emergency services at Harbor. Some days only one or two beds were available in the state hospital, and one or two beds per day, some days, were available elsewhere to cope with that overwhelming mass of sick people.

I had occasion to write about my job experience in a local psychiatric newsletter last year and what follows is taken from that statement.

Notes From A Chairman And A Deputy Director, May 1983.

A flattering job offer came through the mail the other day. In declining to be considered, I summarized my reasons as follows: "My current job is too wonderful to abandon and too terrible to inflict on anyone else." If nothing else, I think I have learned a fair bit since coming to Los Angeles to undertake my mixed academic and public post on June 8, 1978, the day before Proposition 13 was enacted. On the day after my arrival, a two million dollar psychiatric improvement package for Harbor-UCLA Medical Center promised by Governor Jerry Brown disappeared forever. Within a week, I was preparing the first of what have been six major budget cut recommendations in five years as part of my responsibility as coastal region director for the Los Angeles County Mental Health Department.

Fortunately, love is mostly irrational, and I do love equally and fervently both parts of my job, the professor and chairman duties at Harbor-UCLA Medical Center and the county mental health administrator duties. Also my wife and I love L.A., and in a way, wish we had come here in the 1950's as my medical school classmate, the late Dr. Sheldon Selesnick, was urging. I am in awe of the freeways which in an hour can take one anywhere to share the creative products and energies of this splendid three percent of America (L.A. County's 7 1/2 million population). And I love living on the ocean where it is always cool in the morning and evening, and where I have discovered that the lady fish of the barracuda, sea bass, and halibut family produce a magnificent roe. Last but not least, I find more than a little challenging working with the mental health delivery system of Los Angeles, California. The philosophical goals of our mental health department were well stated by philosopher Harold Taylor: "When all is said and done, the purpose of it all—medicine, literature, art, government, philosophy, law, religion, psychiatry, is to provide the deepest and richest psychological and spiritual life for the greatest number of people." For a true to life other side of the story, see the movie, "Raging Bull."

The job blend, being "chairman and professor" for 25 residents in psychiatric training and an administrator, trying to assure equity and the availability of psychiatric resources for poor people living in a catchment of 2.2 million people does provide some conflicting moments. Still, I have felt for a long time that the greatest challenge in medical education is that of inspiring professionals to feel personally responsible for the quality of our American health care systems. In particular, it is difficult to bring together the efforts of the private, academic, and public sectors in psychiatry, even though the needs of our patients, their families, and our own self interest as well would be served by the power of a unified professional stance. In psychiatry, we create many individual pearls but not enough necklaces.

That's what I'm most proud of at Harbor-UCLA Medical Center, the attempt to create a necklace, one with strands of academic pearls, the fools' gold of promised funding, and the hard rock of cost-per-unit-of-service. The task is not an easy one. We suffer all the problems that come with serving very sick patients with shrinking resources (30% less in 1984 than we had in 1979!). We'd not survive at Harbor as an academic program without the strong personal support of the leaders of the Los Angeles County Mental Health Department. chaired by Dr. John Richard Elpers, and we would not be able to carry out our desperately needed public responsibilites without the support of the department of psychiatry at UCLA led by Drs. L. J. West and Milton Greenblatt. Most of all, it is the commitment of the teachers and residents at Harbor to serve the public patient kindly and well that has allowed us to accomplish what has been a remarkable level of success in reestablishing quality in the Los Angeles County public system in spite of everything.

At Harbor we provide the only psychiatric emergency room services for public patients in our region. (Coastal region's 2.2 million people constitute one percent of America!) In total, some 7,000 people per year, many of them psychotic, come or are brought by police and families to our emergency services for care. For a long time, we weren't very proud of what we could do. Once—in 1980— our young doctors went on strike for a day to protest the abysmal working conditions and the terrible limitations on the care that they could give to their patients. There was a lot of talk at that time about opting out, involving the media, making things so bad that "they" would do something about our situation. After we figured out that there was not any "they" except ourselves, we went on to build, together with nursing, social work, and psychologist colleagues, a really wonderfully improved emergency care system at Harbor, and in the coastal region, one that really does us proud. We built a triage center, a crisis resolution center, and we established strong linkages with other public and community non-hospital programs. We worked to establish some "alternatives to hospitalization," and shortened hospital stays by instituting treatment within hours after the patient arrived. We involved families and friends within the first hours of care. We did our best to prioritize. We did our best.

I need to add that the third piece of the Harbor-UCLA system, the contributions of our consulting psychiatrists and psychologists from the private sector, are vital parts of our programs. These generous and skilled members of our clinical faculty bring a broad and varied perspective about patients and practice that's especially important in a system like ours that has so much emphasis on the very sick patient. Our clinical faculty, numbering almost 75 men and women, donate their expertise to the academic and, thus, the public system.

My job is difficult, and there are times when I think the complexities of the responsibilities are more than I would wish to sustain for very many years. And there is my sense of guilt with regard to the trainees, that too much is being asked of them. However, most of our trainees tell me that their experience at Harbor has been rich and rewarding. And, we on the faculty do everything we can to make it clear that we believe they are a very special group who learn while providing desperately needed services for deeply troubled people. I'm very proud of them. In Los Angeles, more and more, we provide state of the art therapy for many patients in the public system because of the partnership between public, private, and academic psychiatry.

Discussion

Of course, the model of professor-commissioner is not a new one. And there are many examples in contemporary American psychiatry of university "catchments." There are also many examples of university-state hospital linkages.   What is somewhat unique in the Los Angeles situation is the "high stakes" nature of the enterprise.   I am responsible for public mental health funds that total 35 million dollars annually.   Part of that funding buys beds in the state hospital system; some supports academic trainees who provide public service; other portions support professorial stipends of teachers who supervise the public work of student trainees.   Some of our resources are invested in the private sector, and there are many private contractors wishing to bid for "service contracts."   There are regular requests by resident psychiatric physicians for higher pay for their "moonlighting work," i.e., services performed after "regular resident duty hours."   There is a complex problem of negotiating with the residents what constitutes "regular duty" and what might be otherwise compensable.   There are occasional conflict of interest charges both by those who feel that too much of our resources are being invested in the university affiliated hospital, or conversely, those who insist that too much is being diverted from desperately needed hospital care into "useless community programs," etc.   But, on balance, our system seems to work fairly well.

The creation of a trusting, mutually respectful relationship between academic faculty and the public system administrators has produced a variety of bilateral "fringe benefits" that have evolved over time.   For example, a painful administrative question concerning the adequacy of performance of a physician working in a public hospital was skillfully managed by an "academic" consultant, one who knew the hospital and was respected by its staff because of his "academic work" in the public arena.   Conversely, when the California legislature in 1982 instructed the state department of mental health to study the prevalence of physical illness in patients coming for care in the state mental hospital, a portion of the research assignments came to staff at the Harbor-UCLA Medical Center, primarily Professors Jambur Ananth and Annette Brodsky.   Our portion of the study will determine the prevalence of undiagnosed and undetected organic conditions among state hospital patients, the degree to which these conditions caused or exacerbate psychiatric symptoms, and the effectiveness of medical treatment in eliminating psychiatric symptoms.   Patients undergo an exhaustive physical examination, neurologic examination, extensive laboratory investigation, psychometric testing, EKG, EEG and, if appropriate, CAT scan. The results will yield information on undetected medical illness, barriers to treatment, the scope of problems with psychotropic drugs, and a variety of clinical, administrative and other matters of the greatest interest to an academic psychiatry department. The opportunity to participate in this important research project is a special bonus for our staff, one that became available because of the breadth of "academic interests" of the faculty at Harbor.

Conclusion

There truly is a need for psychiatrists to consider our professional priorities. Above all, we need to decide whether we are a "we" and if so, what we (together) are going to do about it.

REFERENCES

1. Rand A: Fountainhead. Indianapolis, Bobbs-Merrill 1943

2. Rand A: Atlas Shrugged. New York, Random House 1957

3. Menninger K: The Crime of Punishment. New York Press, 1966

4. Menninger W: You and Psychiatry. New York, Charles Scribner's Sons, 1948

5. Talbott J: The Death of the Asylum: A critical study of state hospital management, services, and care. New York, Grune & Stratton, 1978

6. Greenblatt M: Psychopolitics. New York, Grune & Stratton, 1978

STATE-UNIVERSITY COLLABORATION:
VIEW FROM BOTH SIDES OF THE BRIDGE

Milton Greenblatt, M.D.

Among the several minority groups that I belong to, probably the one that pleases me the most is a tiny group of American psychiatrists who have tasted life both in the university, as well as in the state hospitals.

In both of these settings, I have had the unforgettable experience of serving in executive or administrative roles.

I have learned not only that survival is possible, but also that such work is fun and to share with you some reflections from 43 years in the psychiatric arena.

During approximately 23 years at the Massachusetts Mental Health Center, we participated in a rich variety of social research and therapeutic programs. Studies of patient and staff interactions on the ward, custodial versus therapeutic programs, and research on executive roles and constellations seemed to lead naturally into an interest in other therapeutic systems (1-12).

As the Massachusetts Mental Health Center grew in all its various endeavors, soon bulging at its seams, its director, Dr. Harry Solomon, announced an interest in collaborating for mutual benefit with a state hospital — the Metropolitan State Hospital. It was arranged that some residents in their second year of training could spend one day a week on one of the "godforsaken" wards to learn what life was like in the "snake pits," and to develop by any means at their disposal, a better and more therapeutic program for patients. Such a rotation was considered at that time, a rather bold experiment in psychiatric education. The wards chosen housed about 70 chronic custodial patients with very, very few staff. Two residents who selected that experience were Gerry Klerman and Ed Sachar. I know of no evidence that this strange experience harmed their subsequent professional careers.

At about the same time, the Russell Sage Foundation supported a multi-hospital program of studies and demonstrations at three different hospitals — Massachusetts Mental Health Center, Metropolitan State Hospital, and the Bedford Veterans Administration Hospital. The results of numerous experiments in social treatment were later reported at length in the book, From Custodial to Therapeutic Patient Care in Mental Hospitals (1955) (13). This book helped significantly to catalyze the national effort to eliminate the new prevailing evils of custodialism — seclusion, wet sheet packs, chemical restraints, physical restraints, and forced feeding.

Moreover, it called attention to the real evils behind punitive, restrictive practices — <u>over routinization, emphasis on procedure rather than person, lack of interest in and knowledge concerning the patients' feelings, and lack of motivation in serving the basic psychological, as contrasted with the physiological, needs of patients.</u>

These explorations in social therapy demonstrated not only that a university department of psychiatry could open up vast opportunities for systems research and system change that were of benefit to its own research organization; they also showed that collaborative demonstrations of social change by university and state, or by university and Veterans Administration, together could fuel a spirit of adventure and creativity in the several hospitals involved. Noteworthy was the fact that a great foundation, dedicated almost exclusively to social research, divined that the social sciences could have a major contribution in improving the therapeutic climate and efficacy of mental hospitals.

Other evidence of successful collaboration between the university and state hospitals, relatively unusual for those times, was a large study of comparative efficacy of electroconvulsive therapy, MAO inhibitors, and tricyclics, involving over 300 patients with various forms of depression, hospitalization at Metropolitan, Medfield, Westborough, and Boston State Hospitals (14). In this study we learned how eager the state hospital personnel were to collaborate in a joint venture in which they were true partners.   Not a little of the success was due to the sensitive and understanding leadership of George Grosser, Ph.D., who possessed a rare understanding and feeling for the extraordinary burdens of patient care carried by state hospital personnel under difficult circumstances.

In two other major studies, Massachusetts Mental Health Center showed considerable interest in the patients of other hospitals insofar as transferring chronic schizophrenic patients from these hospitals to Massachusetts Mental Health Center to demonstrate whether a period of hospitalization in an intensive treatment environment could be beneficial to these so-called chronic, "hopeless" schizophrenics (15,16).

In 1963, I took over the superintendency of Boston State Hospital from the eminent Dr. Walter E. Barton. The contrast between Massachusetts Mental Health Center and Boston State Hospital (BSH) was staggering (17).

The state hospital had 56 buildings compared to four buildings at the university center and:

Twelve times as many patients (2,400 to 200);

One M.D. for every 60 patients, compared to one for every two patients;

One staff person at BSH for every five at Massachusetts Mental Health Center, with most of the state hospital staff in housekeeping and management rather than direct patient care;

The admission rate per annum at BSH was twice that of the university hospital;

Many alcoholic, medical and surgical, geriatric and retarded patients, compared to few or none at the university hospital;

Forty percent of the state hospital population was elderly, compared to none in the university center;

Eighty percent of the state hospital population was custodial, compared to none in the university center;

Hundreds of deaths occurred at the state hospital per year, with rare deaths at the university center;

On the other hand, the per diem costs were five times greater in the university center than in the state hospital,

The patients at the state hospital were poorer, more deteriorated, more difficult to treat, and more deficient in family and other support networks critical to their recovery.

What Were The Implications?

1. Affluence and poverty existed side-by-side, a terrible indictment of our American system, which speaks of equal rights, human rights, and features in its Constitution, guarantees of "equal protection" (14th Admendment), and prohibition of "cruel and unusual punishment" (5th Amendment).

2. The university hospital existed as such only by virtue of its "dumping privileges" upon the state hospital. Cases labelled "chronic," "poor teaching material," or "indequate for the mission" of the teaching hospital could easily be transferred to the state hospital.

In effect, the teaching program of the university center denied the residents and other students contact with many of the basic realities of clinical psychiatry—namely, geriatric, retarded, drug dependent, alcoholic, and chronic patients, in favor of patients who were younger, preferably female, educated, verbally productive, and relatively responsive to treatment.

3. The university hospital transferred all its rejects to the state hospital; expected the state hospital to take care of its dirty linen (literally); and then branded the state hospital as a place of inferior patient care, poor training programs, and poorly motivated staff.

4. The implications with regard to professional role, ideology, and social conscience were even more important.

Outrage and injustice permeated the feelings of the state hospital staff, who felt the university hospital was training snobbish, "cream puff" psychiatrists with little or no appreciation of the role that the state hospital played in serving the poor of the Commonwealth and in making it possible for the university to run an elite, affluent training center.

Denial, guilt, and attempts at self-justification permeated the feelings of the unversity staff when confronted with the contrasts. They rarely, if ever, visited the state hospital.

Nevertheless, this particular state hospital had somehow succeeded in developing for psychiatric and other professionals, training programs in collaboration with two Boston medical schools — Boston University and Tufts. In addition, several research programs as well as innovative treatment demonstrations were making use of the rich and varied clinical population — a population in many ways richer and more varied than that in the university center.

Over the years, the university hospital had become more and more selective of its cases. It had become a favorite place for admitting college students with acute mental disorders. In such a setting, many psychiatric residents were naturally inclined to choose a life of psychoanalytically-oriented office practice with little feeling of responsibility for the welfare of the larger community.

But all this changed dramatically following the Joint Commission Report (18), and the introduction of the deinstitutionalization movement, based on leadership provided by President Kennedy, the National Institute of Mental Health, the American Psychiatric Association, and dozens of other interested groups. Some stroke of fortune placed me in the commissioner's seat in Massachusetts at this particular time, with a legislative mandate for a sweeping reorganization of the whole mental health treatment system of the Commonwealth.

The Reorganization Act of 1966 (19) assigned to the Massachusetts Mental Health Center a specific geographic catchment area of 210,000 people, with the mandate to provide services to all the citizens in the area, excluding no category of disease, age, ethnic, or racial group. Boston State Hospital also was assigned a catchment area. Transfer of cases from one catchment area to another — from Massachusetts Mental Health Center to Boston State Hospital — was frowned upon and finally ceased. The pattern of cases admitted to Massachusetts Mental Health Center changed dramatically: elderly, drug-addicted, and retarded patients were accepted. New community programs were developed to meet the challenge of caring for a total population. The changeover was not easy.

Boston State Hospital's metamorphosis was even more remarkable. In 1963, the hospital population was 2,400. Over the next two decades, the population declined to less than 100 patients hospitalized. In 1963, the outpatient service had about 200 patients. Now, many hundreds of patients are in ambulatory care. Buildings on the campus are used for a variety of other purposes, including use as transitional centers for the Department of Correction and Youth Service Board. The immense burden of taking care of too many patients with too few staff has been greatly relieved.

After World War II, Medfield State Hospital affiliated with Boston University, Fernald State School with the neurological service of Massachusetts General Hospital, and Lindemann Mental Health Center with the psychiatric program of the Massachusetts General Hospital.

As new mental health centers were developed throughout the state, we tried wherever possible to relate them to general hospitals and to institutions of higher learning. In a state rich in schools and colleges, this seemed the natural way to go. Advice to superintendents of the new mental health centers was to cultivate the goodwill and cooperation of students and faculties of educational facilities, encourage volunteering, stimulate educational programs, sponsor joint research projects, and develop a climate of clinical innovation, emphasizing the therapeutic possibilities of community-based facilities and support systems.

Of all the projects that characterized that early period of cooperation between university hospital and state facility, perhaps the most gratifying was the student volunteer movement. Undergraduates from Harvard and Radcliffe, and later several other colleges or universities in the area, with a little encouragement and guidance from senior professionals from both Massachusetts Mental Health Center and the state hospital, undertook to transform the drab and lonely atmosphere of the state hospital wards into a more friendly and humane environment. Conceiving many ways to approach patients and make their lives more meaningful, they practiced what they called "friendship therapy," which was based on making a close and enduring relationship with chronic patients. Their efforts were remarkably successful in returning many of these patients to the community, or at least making their existence more interesting.

Not only did they bring to the hospital their youth, enthusiasm, and optimism, but they also developed several halfway houses, provided a summer vacation home on Cape Cod for a number of back-ward patients, engaged the interest of their instructors from the colleges and universities, and wrote a book about their experiences (20).

Thus, the state-university collaboration demonstrated how it is possible to mobilize vast reserves of high quality manpower on behalf of the mentally ill — without expenditure of new funds. Further, not only did patients benefit, but students learned a great deal. Not infrequently they changed their plans, deciding in favor of a career in some aspect of mental health — so great was the recognition of need for their services, and the resultant gratification of becoming meaningful to a less fortunate person.

In 1965, having worked on both sides of the divide, we wrote:

> "It has been apparent for some time that great gains could be made toward solving the problems facing the embattled state hospitals, if university centers would take the lead and develop the means of bridging the gap between their centers and the state mental hospitals. It is also clear, but not so apparent, that the university centers, far from losing status, prestige, or training strength by such a collaboration, might, in fact, add to their stature." (21)

In the present fiscal climate, many university hospitals are finding it necessary to change the mix of cases in favor of those who can pay. Also, hospitalization time is being reduced by third-party payers, making long-term relationships between trainees and patients difficult. The state hospitals, however, offer a very rich assortment of clinical material, particularly lower socio-economic cases, long-term cases, and more freedom to explore long-term relationships. Earlier assumption of ward responsibility is generally possible for psychiatric trainees. The case sample helps residents gain a broader and more valid view of the community's real problems; at the same time, they learn how patients are handled in a system that is very different from the ivory tower from which they may emanate (22). Good or bad, it is a system for which all of us, as citizens, are ultimately responsible.

REFERENCES

1.   Kegeles SS, Hyde RW, Greenblatt M: Sociometric network on an acute psychiatric ward.   Group Psychotherapy, 5: 91-110, 1952

2.   Hyde RW, Greenblatt M, Boyd R: Authority in attendant-patient relationships.   J Ner Ment Dis, 117: 166, 1953

3.   Morimoto FR, Greenblatt M: Personnel awareness of patients' socializing capacity. Am J Psychiatry, 110: 443-447, 1953

4.   Morimoto FR, Baker TS, Greenblatt M: Similarity of socializing interests as a factor in selection and rejection of psychiatric patients.   J Ner Ment Dis, 120: 56-61, 1954

5.   Boyd R, Baker T, Greenblatt M: Ward social behavior: an analysis of patient interaction at highest and lowest extremes.   Nursing Research, 3: 77-80, 1954

6.   Boyd RW, Kegeles SS, Greenblatt M: Outbreak of gang destructive behavior on a psychiatric ward. J Ner Ment Dis 120: 338-342, 1954

7.   Greenblatt M, York RH, Brown EL: From Custodial to Therapeutic Patient Care in Mental Hospitals. New York, Russell Sage Foundation, 1955

8.   Hyde RW, Greenblatt M, Wells FL: The role of the attendant in authority and compliance: notes on ten cases. Genet Psychol, 54: 107-126, 1956

9.   Wells FL, Greenblatt M, Hyde RW: As the Psychiatric Aide Sees His Work and Problems. Genetic Psychology Monographs, 53: 3-73, 1956

10.   Greenblatt M, Levinson DJ, Williams RH (eds):   The Patient and the Mental Hospital. Glencoe, Ill, Free Press, 1957

11. Umbarger CC, Morrison AP, Dalsimer JS, et al: College Students in a Mental Hospital. Prepared with the assistance and supervision of Kantor D, Greenblatt M. New York, Grune & Stratton, 1962

12. Hodgson RC, Levinson DJ, Zaleznik A: The Executive Role Constellation. Cambridge, Harvard Business School, Divison of Research, 1965

13. Greenblatt M, York R, Brown EL: From Custodial to Therapeutic Patient Care in Mental Hospitals. New York, Russell Sage Foundation, 1955

14. Greenblatt M, Grosser GH, Wechsler H: Differential response of hospitalized depressed patients to somatic therapy. Am J Psychiatry, 120: 935-943, 1964

15. Greenblatt M (Ed.): Drugs in Combination With Other Therapies. New York, Grune & Stratton, 1975

16. Grinspoon L, Ewalt JR, Shader RI: Schizophrenia: Pharmacotherapy and Psychotherapy. Baltimore, Williams & Wilkins, 1972

17. Greenblatt M: University-hospital collaboration in psychiatric education. Hosp Community Psychiatry, 16: 167-169, 1965

18. Joint Commission on Mental Illness and Health: Action for Mental Health: Final Report of the Joint Commission on Mental Illness and Health. New York, Basic Books, 1961

19. Commonwealth of Massachusetts Comprehensive Mental Health and Mental Retardation Services Act, December 1966

LESSONS LEARNED:

WHAT WORKS AND DOESN'T WORK, AND HOW TO OVERCOME RESISTANCES

John A. Talbott, M.D.

Milton Greenblatt, M.D.

From both the review of the existing literature and the examples given in the subsequent chapters, several important lessons can be learned concerning what works and what doesn't work to make state-university collaborations successful.   In this chapter, we will discuss what seems to work, what does not work, and how to overcome obstacles or resistances.   We have chosen to group items differently within each larger section and hope this approach will not overly confuse the reader.

What Works

1. Strong and committed leadership.   Probably the most important single ingredient to the success of state-university collaborations is strong and committed leadership on both sides.   As we have seen from almost all the examples, it is very helpful to have leaders from both the university and public hospital who are optimistic, persistent knowledgeable, and even charismatic.   In addition, it is important that they present good role models to the trainees, as well as the faculty of the university department of psychiatry and the staff of the state hospital.

Two common errors are the assumptions that: 1) verbal support necessarily means specific action, and 2) support early in the project means support throughout the project.   What we look for from the key leadership is not just a commitment to the concept of state-university collaboration, and belief that it will result in mutual payoffs, but mainly the willingness to accompany the theoretical endorsement with an appropriate commitment of resources undiminished over time.

Practically, this means that not only must numerous frank and open meetings take place between the involved parties, but there must be a recognition that staff support will have to be assiduously cultivated in both systems, and that progress will be reveiwed both at regular intervals as well as on an as-needed basis, to resolve problems as they arise.

It is apparent from reading the reports of successful collaborations such as those in Maryland, Oregon, and North Carolina, that positive committed leadership was a hallmark of their relationships.   One of the problems in assessing this ingredient is that the authors of the chapters are too modest to fully acknowledge this factor fully.

2.   Personal attitudes and attributes. Also of critical importance are the personal attitudes and attributes of the key individuals involved in the collaboration, e.g., the training director(s), service chief(s), discipline head(s), in addition to the key leadership. Programs are most successful when all of these individuals are positive, optimistic, trusting, enthusiastic, expectant, flexible, and creative. It also helps if they are excited rather than discouraged by the challenge of the collaboration and if they see the project opening up a bigger world than exists at present.

Again, the reports of the successful joint ventures document that when all concerned entered into the program with a "can-do" attitude, progress ensued.

3.   Joint nature of the collaboration. Collaborations appear to be most successful when they are based on the perception that both parties' needs will be satisfied, and when there are trade-offs that appear equitable to both sides (e.g., training sites for stipends). In addition, it is helpful if the two sides have a similar set of values, goals, and views of the solutions to the attendant problems. Finally, in implementing the actual training, administration, service, or research programs, the designation of "bridging persons" who have joint appointments increases communication, trust, and resultant success.

The collaboration may be significantly advanced if these "bridging persons" include at least one or more individuals who have worked in the state system and know its realities. Further, those who have proven themselves in both cultures - university and state system - will quickly gain the confidence of both sides.

The validity of the principle of "jointness" is demonstrated in looking at the mutuality of needs of the participants in North Carolina, the mutuality of purpose of the Maryland planners, the joint goals in

Pennsylvania, the joint bodies that carried out the program in Oregon, and the joint appointments and to and fro activities of the faculty and staff in Maryland.

4.   Program design.   Most successful programs emphasize the importance of high quality supervision and teaching, close communication and cooperation, and exposure of trainees to a wide variety of patients, experiences, and settings. In addition, they avoid excessive service burdens and minimize scheduling or transportation problems.   Finally, they merge the existing separate programs into an integrated one.

A further feature of a successful long-term collaboration will be the adequate supervision of residents that accomplishes at least three objectives: 1) teaching the elements of individual patient care and treatment, 2) understanding the workings of the state institutions, and 3) assisting the residents to endure the frustrations of practicing psychiatry in a less than perfect environment.

It is highly desirable that state hospital personnel be involved in teaching and supervising the university residents, and vice versa - if the state hospital has its own program. Appointments of state hospital personnel to teaching positions in the university may be a sine qua non. If such appointments are not possible, then every attempt should be made to hire well-trained university graduates on the staff of the state facility. Part-time arrangements may be feasible as a first step. Also recommended is the appointment of a pair of university members to state hospitals positions at the same time. Research, as well as our own experience, confirms that such pairing results in mutual support that permits longer tenure and greater success in overcoming obstacles, than working alone in the new setting.

Here again, we can see in the design of successful programs, elements such as clear division of responsibility between service and education in Maryland or emphasis on both curricular and experiential factors in Oregon. Both programs used their best faculty and provided high quality experiences, teaching, and supervision.

5. <u>Systems factors</u>. Several ingredients in successful programs comprise what can best be termed as systems factors. These include: the past experiences in collaborative efforts on the part of both parties; the similarities and differences in demography of faculty, trainees, and patients; the geographic and cultural proximity of both institutions; the labeling and perception of the new collaboration as "special"; the advantage if both parties are "public" institutions; budgetary flexibility, e.g., the use of contracts rather than line items; and the diversity and interdigitation of jobs, experiences, and settings.

A variety of other systems factors should also be mentioned, including: the provision of a private office and adequate secretarial support for university faculty working in a state setting; the involvement of university personnel in the social life of the state hospital to understand better its problems and values, as well as to deepen collegial relationships and encourage friendships; and access to policy-making bodies and decision-makers to learn how the specific state institution relates to the overall state system with its legal and budgetary constraints, standard and rate setting missions, and demands and expectations of its community.

Maryland had a history of attempts at collaboration; Oregon and Alberquerque were the only shows in town, and North Carolina offered geographic proximity and the impending reality of putting in only one NIMH training grant. In addition, all involved public-public collaboration and clearly saw themselves as special and ground-breaking.

6. <u>Success and money</u>. Finally, one of the most important predictors of future success is past success - e.g., "success breeds success." Thus, while money is the catalyst that often enables the collaboration to go forward, money alone is insufficient. Planners must ensure a sufficient number of small gains and payoffs for each party for success to continue.

A common question confronting beginning participants is whether the collaboration needs new money or can
go forward through the flexible use of old money. This is
where imaginative administration is required, particularly
since nowadays new monies are harder and harder to come
by. A critical analysis of the current utilization of
resources is in order. A great administrator, Harry C.
Solomon, used to extoll the virtues of such mundane
administrative techniques as scrounging, making do,
muddling through, innovating, and nagging.   Since any
signficant systems change invokes resistance from some
quarter or another, patience and persistence may be the
paramount elements of success at some critical junctures.

In Oregon and Maryland, success was built upon
success, and in North Carolina attitudes gradually shifted
more and more positively. Money was clearly a catalyst in
New Mexico, but in Maryland, no new funding was used.

What Doesn't Work

To some considerable extent, the following represent
the opposite side of the coin of what works; e.g., if
optimism and positive attitudes work, then pessimism and
negative attitudes do not.

1. Weak leadership. If the key leadership is weak,
   divided, or negative about the collaborative efforts,
   it may well fail. If the leaders are out of step with
   the rest of the faculty, staff, or trainees, collaboration may be extremely difficult. And if the leaders
   of the two parties do not see eye to eye on a variety
   of issues, share common goals and values, or have
   widely divergent personality styles, it will certainly
   be tough sledding.

Our authors are discreet in avoiding too much finger-
pointing, but in Georgia it appears that the leadership
change had a drastic effect on the intended collaborative
effort, and in New York, leadership undermined the best of
plans.

2. Negative attitudes. Likewise, in unsuccessful
   collaborations, there is frequently a high degree of
   mistrust on both sides, fueled by fears of
   exploitation, control, or constraints on funding.

Myths or stereotypic notions about both "academics" and "administrators" may impede progress, and previous bad experiences, even with different leaders, may poison the water.

Two negative attitudes on the part of the university, frequently highlighted by the authors in this book, are that oftentimes the university representatives: 1) act like they are bringing enlightenment to the state hospital - a very denigrating attitude, almost sure to invite rejection of the project by the state hospital personnel; and 2) treat the members of the state hospital staff as if they are not experts in any area of psychiatry and therefore have nothing to teach the university's residents or faculty. Such attitudes fail to consider that state hospital professionals have amassed a vast clinical experience, often with clinical issues not seen in the university setting. Further, state staff understand the realities of working very hard with fewer personnel and resources than the university faculty generally enjoy and treat some of the very toughest patients, including those rejected by the university as not conforming to its "training mission."
On the other hand, state hospital personnel may have other anxieties and concerns, such as a fear that the university really aims to take over part or all of the state institution for its own benefit, e.g., to augment its patient pool, to gain space for more laboratories and research, or to latch onto state hospital salaries for expansion of university faculty. "Where will I fit in?" they ask, "Are my days numbered?" State hospital personnel may feel that the university faculty members are "spoiled" by the advantages they enjoy, that research and teaching careers constitute a "soft life," and that university training programs create "cream puff" psychiatrists, ill equipped to function in the reality in which the state personnel work. Such attitudes too, lead to contempt and suspicion, weakening chances of alliances.
In Utah, the lack of understanding and mutual rebuffing was destructive to the development of a productive collaboration; in Georgia, a shift in leadership orientation undermined what was already a shaky situation; in both California and Georgia, antimedical attitudes were destructive; in New York the exact opposite of Maryland's effort to improve working conditions occurred; and in California and Ohio, distrust and divergent priorities helped doom the programs.

3.   Financial factors. While we stated that money was
     not in and of itself enough to guarantee the
     collaboration's success, financial issues may well
     doom it. For instance, too short-term a commitment
     may threaten a cohort of trainees' future years;
     unanticipated budget cuts may constrict either
     educational or service programs; financial disincen-
     tives may put off collaborative overtures; and
     unstable governmental funding may frighten medical
     school or university administrators.

The clearest example of money becoming a problem
in collaborative efforts occurred in New York City's
hospitals where charges were made of exploitation and
abuse of contract funding.

4.   Vested interests. A major obstacle to implement-
     ing successfull state-university collaborations is
     posed by the individual parties' vested interests. This
     may generate disputes over turf, especially regarding
     who is responsible for what, and clashes regarding
     commitments to buildings versus programs.

Vested interests in California resulted in each party
both "going its own way" and ignoring formal arrangements
as well as past history. In North Carolina, while territorial
concerns as well as those of a "take-over," surfaced
initially, they were successfully worked through.

5.   Deficiences in state facilities. Where state
     facilities are substandard, these deficiencies may
     hamper successful collaborations. For instance, uni-
     versity programs may balk at collaborations with
     facilities whose staff is poorly-trained and possesses
     a low morale; or whose major interest in affiliation is
     to solve some of their monumental service demands;
     or when there are abysmal working conditions and
     very poor quality patient care; or an exceptionally
     rigid bureaucracy.

Poor working conditions were the primary target of
the Maryland planners, but in Utah, state officials found no
way of working around them. In Georgia, on the other
hand, the deficiencies involved a drastic shift in policy and
lack of support for previously stated intentions.

6.   Programmatic problems. State-university collaborations also have a history of not working optimally, when trainees' rotations are merely token or seen as second-class, when there are other higher-status "tracks," where lower-status faculty are assigned, where trainees' roles are narrow, rotations are unifocal, supervision is supplied by non-psychiatrists or paraprofessionals, or when there are insufficient opportunities to follow patients over long periods of time.

In Utah, clinical burdens prevented adequate attention to other priorities, and in California, constraints on the program from both sides slowly choked it.

7.   System factors.   Frequently, there are adverse elements in the environment in which either the university or state hospital operate.   These include such factors as extreme fragmentation of services, more grossly inadequate funding than is common in public systems, and large geographic distances. Since individual states have differing funding commitments to their state hospital systems and these fluctuate over time, the state of any system's governmental commitment at any particular time, is also important.

Clearly the shift in orientation in Georgia and Sacramento signalled the demise of their well-intentioned collaborations.

Overcoming Resistances

It should be clear by now that just as some collaborative efforts fail because of the resistances enumerated above, others succeed because these obstacles have been worked through and surmounted.   We do not contend that all resistance can be overcome, but as optimistic and action-oriented individuals, we believe in trying to tackle those problems that can be tackled.
Some problems, such as weak leadership, can only be remedied by changes in the people occupying the positions.   Others, such as changing key individuals' values, are probably unchangeable.   Yet others, such as vested interests, decrepit buildings, geographical distance, and

overly rigid bureaucracies, can be worked around and changed very gradually over time. However, a host of other resistances can be attacked directly.

1. <u>Negative attitudes.</u> The host of negative attitudinal problems that often hamper effective state–university collaboration can be altered through a variety of means. Since many persons opposed to such activities are opposed because they have never seen a successful program, it is extremely useful to expose them to successful efforts through readings, presentations, and most especially, site visits. In addition, even the most oppositional will often bend if they experience a genuine need (e.g., additional stipends); if the reality rather than the feared is presented; and if they become involved gradually through a joint task-oriented, problem-solving planning effort. Achieving group consensus through such shared experiences is critical, as is an appreciation for proceding in small steps, being persistent, and letting success build on success.

We want to acknowledge that a certain amount of skepticism is natural and inevitable in joining a new enterprise, especially one that tries to join two systems, each under independant management. Positive, optimistic, and enthusiastic attitudes do not arise full blown from the head of Zeus, but often have to be developed or cultivated by the serious exchange of views, together with a study of other systems, including some that have failed and others that have succeeded. At present, such systems studies are usually anecdotal. What is needed is a comparative analysis of a number of such experiments, that teases out more precisely factors that favor success versus those that lead to failure. This kind of research would benefit the field greatly, and we strongly urge the field to undertake such efforts, and the NIMH to fund them.

2. <u>Lack of resource stability.</u> Instability of and uncertainty about funding remains a key obstacle. Often, incentives can be built into an arrangement to make funding more appealing. Writing contracts rather than utilizing state line items offers some protection from yearly fluctuations in support, as does multiple source funding, e.g., from grants, local

government, and third-parties. Commitments made for the duration of training of any one cohort of psychiatric residents or fellows, such as two or four years, also will allay university administrators' anxiety. Finally, specific legislation and a history of good experiences over extended periods of time will help.

3. <u>Low prestige</u>. At the start of one collaboration, the esteemed chairman of a leading academic department of psychiatry "assigned" himself as the first on-site preceptor, and the training program's most outstanding resident, as its first trainee. This action gave a clear message about the status of the collaboration, the high quality of faculty to be selected, the importance of good role models, and the critical nature of the program to the residency experience. Also helpful is a "beefing up" of the quality of the services provided, eliminating excessive service burdens, avoiding different "tracks," and exposing residents and others to a variety of experiences (e.g., inpatient, outpatient, day hospital; forensic, administrative, and adolescent; and community, rehabilitative, and liaison services).

4. <u>Divisiveness</u>. Splits between "us" and "them" can often be narrowed through "joint" activities. These include joint needs' assessments, joint task assignments, and joint problem-solving activities. For example, the Maryland Plan involved persons from both sectors working out on an agreed-upon series of goals, objectives, resource allocations, and implementation steps. Divisiveness is also reduced when each party feels it is getting a fair shake, and the trade-offs appear equal to all concerned.

5. <u>Rigid bureaucracies or hierarchies</u>. Oftentimes, as stated above, these must be accepted and worked around, but it is always helpful for all parties to have adequate knowledge of each others' bureaucractic constraints and limitations, as well as the political savvy to operate within them. It is also useful for them to appreciate the rigidity of their own as well as their counterpart's organization. For instance, it is often eye-opening for state hospital staff to

realize how political and hierarchical the university bureaucracy is. Finally, as with so many other issues, in dealing with bureaucracies, persistence often does pay off in the end.

6.   Lack of a perceived need. Often the state sees no need to become involved with the university. "All they want is our money, what can we possibly get in return?" Likewise, the academic department sees no compelling reason to involve itself in yet another political morass. "Why should we take on more clinical responsibilities, we already have too many beds?" It is only when a genuine needs assessment demonstrates the mutual advantages to each, or the leadership sees the advantages of being involved in the bigger world, that such perceptions shift.

7.   State facility deficiencies. Changing the bricks and mortar of the state hospital may be impossible, but improving other aspects of its functioning may be less formidable, such as hiring better trained clinical staff, improving patient programming, and upgrading community placements. It is conventional wisdom that one only can change factors such as these during the period of negotiation of the collaboration, but it is our experience and conclusion from examining successful programs such as in Maryland, that even after the program has been agreed upon, quality of care and facility deficiencies can be improved.

8.   Resistance to any change. Any new program threatens some persons. There are several generic strategies to overcoming obstacles and implementing change. (1-5) These include:

  - support from above
  - active leadership
  - a critical mass of change agents
  - a clear mandate
  - picking the right time
  - choosing the right place
  - flexibility
  - open communication
  - increasing participation and decreasing central authority

- valuing change itself
- selecting new courses of action
- changing tactics
- disseminating information widely
- attacking on all fronts, and
- encouraging even more change

The use of small pilot efforts, redeployment of staff and faculty, and academic or institutional inducements or rewards is often effective in reducing resistance to state-university collaborations.

Summary

While the literature on implementing state-university collaborations around educational, service, and research activities is spare, the experience is vast. From the examples found in the literature and provided in this book, many lessons can be learned about what brings about successful collaborations and what impedes them. In the final section of this chapter, we have drawn upon our own and various experiences throughout the country in outlining some strategies for combating resistances. Given the shrinking or stabilization of the health care dollar, and the increasing mutual needs of both academic departments and public institutions, such collaborations will prove increasingly important to both parties, and attention to their initiation, nourishment, and growth becomes more critical.

REFERENCES

1. Greenblatt M, York RH, Brown EL: From custodial to therapeutic patient care in mental hospitals. New York, Russell Sage Foundation, 1955

2. Greenblatt M: University-hospital collaboration in psychiatric education. Ment Hosp 16:167-169, 1965

3. Greenblatt M, Sharaf MR, Stone EM: Dynamics of Institutional Change: The Hospital in Transition. Pittsburgh, University Of Pittsburgh Press, 1971

4. Greenblatt M: Psychopolitics. New York, Grune & Stratton, 1978

5. Talbott JA: The Death of the Asylum: A Critical Study of State Hospital Management, Services, and Care. New York, Grune & Stratton, 1978, pp 91-97

EDUCATION FOR COLLABORATION

Carolyn B. Robinowitz, M.D.

Introduction

Graduate education in psychiatry represents a complex interplay of learning experiences: the theoretical exposes all facets of the discipline, including the constantly expanding knowledge in the neurosciences, the understanding of the role of socio-cultural factors on development and illness; the study of efficacy and outcome, and other factors that provide a basis for the biospychosocial science of the field; the "apprenticeship" in which the neophyte psychiatrist learns, through hands-on experience, to diagnose and treat mental disorders, working with both patients and their families, as well as providing indirect care through consultation-liaison models; and the emphasis on education that assists the practitioner to tolerate the uncertainties of the present with sufficient flexibility to adapt to future directions and needs. The first and third statements serve as examples of the core educational approach; the second statement points out the more practical aspect of training. While the terms "graduate education" and "residency training" are often used interchangeably, they exemplify two different approaches to the post-medical school learning experience that, ideally, must be blended in the formation of the psychiatrist.

Historical Context

In the past two decades, the American Psychiatric Association has sponsored two conferences on psychiatric education and practice. Known as "decade" conferences, these meetings have resulted in consensus regarding future directions. Ewalt, in bridging the work of the 1962 and 1974 conferences, noted: "Throughout the training program, the residents should be helped to develop a sense of values as well as clinical proficiency. In final analysis, education and training in clinical psychiatry are designed to give the resident a body of knowledge, certain definite skills, and an attitude toward his work and the responsibility of his profession" (1). While the content and directions of the field have changed, this statement of educational goals remains apt, yet another decade later. At the time of Ewalt's comments, residency programs tended to be divided into university-based or state/community-based, a kind of town-gown dichotomy in which "town" was generally perceived as second class.   The university-based, academic residency tended to provide education for residents in a somewhat rarefied atmosphere.   Unfettered by pressing service needs, the resident worked with carefully chosen "teaching patients" who were treated on special services.   These patients tended to be educated and verbal; their illnesses were of limited severity, such that some were referred to as the "worried well."   The mentor and role model tended to be a highly skilled clinician, whose expertise was in demonstrating phenomenology and psychopathology and whose skills were most viewed in the psychosocial end of the biopsychosocial continuum.   This faculty member was either a privately practicing clinician, often an analyst, whose lifestyle as well as intellectual competence was admired, or a full-time academician with time for thoughtful deliberation and research.   Promotion came through research, not patient care, and federal funds for research and clinical training, not service dollars, supported the department and the resident.

Residents graduating from such programs tended to move quickly into clinical practice, emulating their charismatic professors.   While many chose to work initially (at least part-time) in salaried positions in the public sector, they tended to leave within a year or two, citing the difficulties of the public sector as a work site. (2,3) While in some cases, "recent graduates" private practices had become sufficiently built up to provide adequate income, many of these young psychiatrists reported feeling inadequately trained to care for the patients or deal with the problems inherent in these settings.

At the same time, there was another setting for training the so-called world of clinical care, very separate from the rarefied air of the academic department of psychiatry.   The public hospital was the last resort of the less fortunate patient, who was felt to be too sick, uneducated or "not sufficiently psychologically minded" to be a good teaching case. There, psychiatry residents often received a more second-class education.   Many were foreign nationals, with sufficient language difficulties or lack of exposure to local culture that they could not really understand what their patients were saying (verbally or symbolically).   There was a shortage of faculty, and residents seemed to exist more to provide service than to receive training or education, with service needs taking precedence over residents' educational needs. Their patient loads were so large that there simply wasn't sufficient time to study patients in detail; thus, learning was pragmatic and not always transferable to other situations. Faculty, too, were overwhelmed by large caseloads and limited time, and many faculty had little opportunities for their own professional development, nor did they have experiences in learning how to teach or supervise. Further, many residents had only limited licenses to practice, and even more limited self-confidence, and thus maintained their dependency (occasionally hostile) on the system, in spite of being exploited. While this description represents an extreme, the extremes existed all too often.

Most historians recognize that this separation of the university and the community was a result of the changes initiated in response to the Flexner Report. Medical training moved from an on-the-job apprenticeship to a complex and reproducible system of experiences in educational institutions. This change enriched the academic institutions, leading to the integration of research in education and practice, but in part, at the expense of the community hospital and its patients (even though eventually, these patients profited from the scientific advances originating in the medical schools).

While Flexner initiated a revolution in medical education, the social changes of the seventies and the fiscal changes of the eighties, with their resultant changes in service delivery, also have initiated a major change in medical education and practice. The extent of their impact remains to be seen. Yet, these changes force us to consider the response to the question, "Teaching, for what?"

Education and Service Delivery

It is an axiom of all education that goals and objectives of educational experiences or programs must be clearly stated, and in advance, if we are to know whether we have accomplished what we have intended. As is often stated, "If you don't know where you're going, you can't know if you got there."

The practice of psychiatry has changed. Psychiatrists are increasingly becoming the mental health professionals caring for the most seriously mentally ill. In these endeavors, they are utilizing advances in the science of psychiatry including psychopharmacology, family therapy, outcome studies, and other approaches to the understanding and treatment of mental disorders.   Patients, even those with the most serious mental illnesses, are more apt to have short hospital stays, with cost constraints resulting from DRG's and deinstitutionalization influencing length of stay.   At the same time, rapid circulation of knowledge has led to more universal approaches to practice, such that the academic scientific advances quickly become translated into routine clinical care.

In all of medicine, there is increasing emphasis on new approaches (or modification of older approaches) to service delivery.   Younger psychiatrists are more apt to work in salaried positions, and fee-for-service practice, although still available and highly valued, is facing strong competition from the organized health care delivery systems.   While psychiatry remains the medical specialty in shortest supply, it has become clear that the need for psychiatrists is greatest in the public sector.   As such, there are real opportunities, not to mention urgent needs, for well-trained psychiatrists to provide leadership and care in the public sector, and particularly in the state mental health system.

As it becomes clear that psychiatry will be practiced in many settings significantly different from the current locales of training, and that the traditional solo, private practice setting will have the fewest vacancies, residents will require exposure to different types of patients with a broader range and severity of illness, from many different social classes and cultural backgrounds, as well as learning to work in different settings with a variety of models of organization and care.   Such an educational program will provide training for the realities of practice in the decade to come.   Additionally, the programs must also provide effective education for the future changes in patient needs and the diversity of practice settings and types of care organization that will emerge in the twenty-first century. They must experience diversity to be prepared for changes which we cannot yet predict.

Several chapters in this volume cite the advantages that can accrue to the academic department of psychiatry from collaboration with state mental health programs, especially emphasizing the financial benefits arising from the contributions provided by the state.   There is no doubt that such funds are important, particularly as federal dollars have decreased to the point of non-existence, and funds for patient care services provided by residents are in jeopardy. Thompson et al noted a decline in the use of state hospitals as training sites. (4) The Maryland situation tends to contradict this finding, although the energy and innovation of the Maryland educational experience is unique. (5) The positive experiences cited earlier in this volume also demonstrate that the state system can be attractive and fulfilling.

Nonetheless, the state sector is a vital part of a good residency program by its addition of a number of patients with the severe disorders that require the nonsubstitutable skills of a psychiatrist. There, faculty can serve as mentors and role-models, recruiting these residents into the public sector. Furthermore, the knowledge and skills gained by residents in these settings will assist in the transition from residents to practitioner, such that the newly graduated residents will be better prepared and more competent and therefore comfortable working with the patients found in such settings.

Collaborative ventures provide the opportunity for bridging the gap between theory and practice, town and gown, and minimizing the stereotypic dichotomy described above. As these programs become innovative ventures, each system gains from the other. Transfer of advances in scientific knowledge to the community will be facilitated. The intellectual excitement of the academic medical center can be found in the research and educational activities initiated in the state system, with resulting improvement of quality of care as well as staff satisfaction. Academic psychiatry too, will become a more reality-oriented setting, adapting to fulfill its educational and research roles in the context of delivering high quality service, as faculty and trainees are exposed to a broader variety of patients and problems.

Educational Needs

Other authors in this volume have emphasized the factors that promote or impede successful collaborative efforts between state and university systems, implying that strong collaboration will lead to good education. While that implication is basically correct, there are some factors that must be considered solely from their educational perspective – how to make the learning experience a strong one for residents, who will be equipped for practice not only in the nineties, but for whatever the future shall bring.

We must avoid teaching residents "what to know" as opposed to "how to think." The former, while technically correct for the moment, does not prepare a professional for practice activities. Rather, a documented concern for ongoing educational efforts, awareness of the need for life–long learning, and an awareness that what we know and how we work is constantly changing, are a base for developing problem–solving approaches, not just technical behaviors.

The first important factor is integration. The state facility must not become the place where the resident rotates for experiences in service delivery, while education and research continue to be emphasized at the "home base" university teaching hospital. Rather, each setting must have a blend and balance of these three functions. While there will be differences in balance, absence of any of the three will make that aspect of the program "second class."

Another important factor is commitment. Program success requires commitment of faculty and administrators alike to ensure adequate priority for educational activities. Since the academic departments that engage in such collaborative out–reach efforts are among the least prestigious in the university (e.g., psychiatry, community and public health), there must be adequte protection of scholarship not only for the sake of current residents, but also for the survival and strength of the department. At the same time, the department must be willing to work with clinicians and administrators in the service setting to improve their educational as well as clinical skills.

Collaborations often are begun in an atmosphere of extreme optimism, an atmosphere which can rapidly turn to pessimism when confronted with the difficulties of everyday functioning, particularly in underfunded, over-worked state settings, as well as with the stress that change brings. Only a strong active (not just theoretical) commitment can maintain the forward movement towards the originally agreed–upon goal.

A third and equally important factor is the actual content of the learning experience. It is well known that the locus of training influences student behavior as much as the content of the training experience (the classic example is the psychosocial approach of a medical student in a surgery rotation as compared to a psychiatry rotation). And it is often tempting to allow the site to determine the actual teaching experiences. Yet, in any collaborative program, much effort must be made to ensure that the content is appropriate and meets the outcome stated in the Special Requirements (Essentials). While these regulations do not list specific curricular items or time allocations, they state broad general principles that must be met. The faculty must review the educational experiences not only topic by topic, but also look at the timing, location, and process. For example, assignment to two or more sites tends to result in more block than longitudinal experiences; in such programs, there must be provision for more long-term follow-up of patients with some consistent and on-going supervision. How do residents assigned "away" participate in more formal didactic exercises? If they "return" to the university campus, is there a message about the quality of education provided in the service setting? Conversely, if more formal educational activities are provided in the state setting, is there sufficient oversight to document their quality? Can formal educational activities be planned that involve a minimum of both travel and isolation from peers and colleagues in the "other" setting?

The training program must include both core learning experiences and electives - the latter can be lost when trainees are exposed to two or more settings for clinical education. As the scientific knowledge base of the field expands, residents must be exposed to some of the sub-specialty areas (e.g., geriatric psychiatry, forensic psychiatry, alcohol and substance abuse), as well as approaches to practice (e.g., organizational consultation, administration, emergency psychiatry, and work with other health and mental health professionals).

The faculty represent both a resource and a challenge. There needs to be careful attention to faculty development, to improve faculty scientific and clinical knowledge as well as educational skills. Continuing education is important not only from the concrete knowledge and skill it imparts, but from the message that support of CME demonstrates - that continuous education is vital to professional function. Programs with resources devoted to on-going faculty and staff education document their commitment to quality education. Further, since often theoretical orientation as well as knowledge and skill tend to relate to the setting in which faculty members work, the program should develop some integrative learning activities for faculty from all training sites, so that each can learn from the other, and teach in the least dogmatic and most empirical and integrative manner. Criteria for promotion and tenure must reflect both this approach to faculty development and the departmental view of high priority to all facets of the teaching program, with rewards for excellence in service delivery and educational approaches, as well as research per se. These latter items emphasize the need for control of the educational program. Such control implies some degree of control - even if jointly or mutually held - of the clinical facility. If some control is lacking, the educational institution assumes a responsibility without the authority to implement it. If trainee/student activities (both education and patient care) are subject to exertnal demands, administrative pressures, and other outside forces, the training program will deteriorate and fail, along with the collaboration. While the administrative and service needs must be recognized and met, the quality of education will determine the ultimate success not only of the training program, but of the future recruitment of well-trained psychiatrists qualified to work in such settings.

Thus, such programs require careful planning with integration not only of service delivery, but of the formal and informal learning experiences that make up a residency, and a commitment from both sectors to outcome through innovation, flexibility, and just plain hard work.

REFERENCES

1. Ewalt J: "Reactor's discussion of the preparatory commission's report on content, methodology, faculty, and environment." In the Working Papers of the 1975 Conference on Education of Psychiatrists. American Psychiatric Association, Washington, D.C., 1976 p 257

2. Ash P, Knesper DJ: "Influences from psychiatric education on subsequent career choice: with special reference to work in state hospitals and the shift to private practice." J Psychiat Ed 5(4):285–294, 1981

3. Chan CH, Astrachan BM: "The first post-residency position: Correlations with training program characteristics." J Psychiat Ed 8(2):75–86, 1984

4. Thompson JW, Checker A, Witkin MJ, et al: "The decline of state mental hospitals as training sites for psychiatric residents." Am J Psychiatry 140(6);704–707, 1983

5. Harbin HT, Weintraub W, Karahasan A, et al: "Psychiatric manpower and public mental health: the Maryland experience." Hosp Community Psychiatry 3:277–281, 1982